Everyday keto

Publications International, Ltd.

Pictured on the front cover *(clockwise from top)*: Bacon-Kale Quiche *(page 237)*, Classic Deviled Eggs *(page 66)* and Mediterranean Steak Salad *(page 130)*.

Pictured on the back cover: Roasted Chicken with Cabbage *(page 98)*.

Photograph on front cover (bottom) and page 130 copyright © Shutterstock.com.

Contributing Writer: Jacqueline B. Marcus, MS, RDN, LDN, CNS, FADA, FAND

ISBN: 978-1-64030-825-1

Manufactured in China.

8 7 6 5 4 3 2 1

Microwave Cooking: Microwave ovens vary in wattage. Use the cooking times as guidelines and check for doneness before adding more time.

Let's get social!

 @Publications_International

 @PublicationsInternational

www.pilcookbooks.com

contents

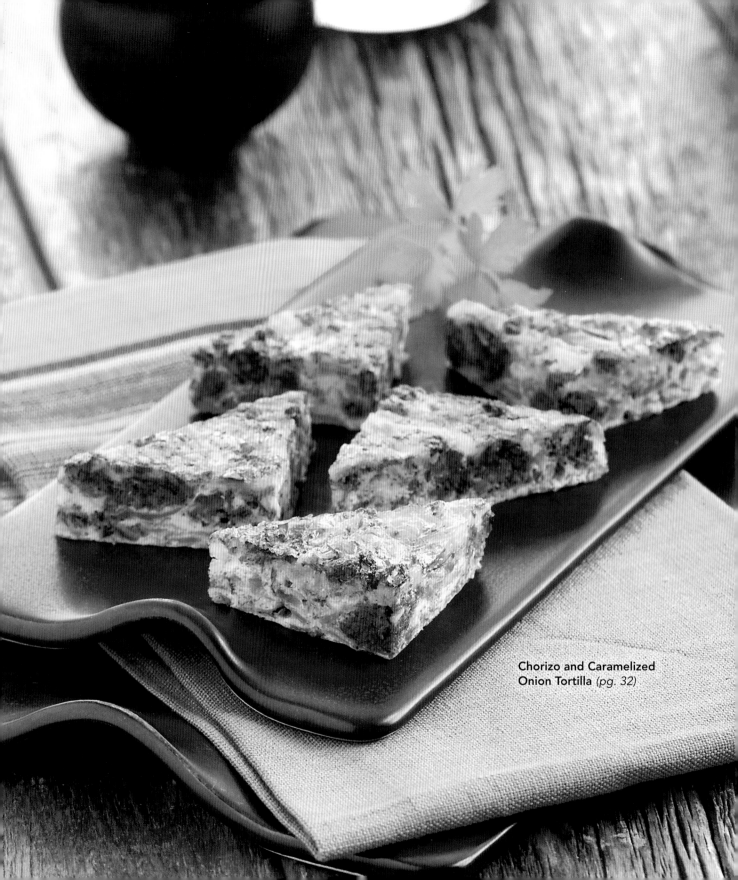

Chorizo and Caramelized
Onion Tortilla (pg. 32)

introduction

Dietary Fats and Oils, Weight and Health

Want to hear some good news about dietary fats and oils—especially how they relate to weight and health?

Consuming dietary fats and oils is not as bad as you might think—nor will consuming dietary fats and oils necessarily make you fat. The right amounts and types of dietary fats and oils may actually be satisfying and contribute to weight loss and weight maintenance. Dietary fats and oils are essential to your overall diet. Understanding what dietary fats and oils are and how they fit into an overall diet will help you with food selection, preparation and meal and menu planning.

The keto diet is based on ketones, organic compounds that are produced when dietary carbohydrates are limited. Ketosis is a normal metabolic process whereby the body burns stored fats instead of glucose from carbohydrates for energy. A diet based on ketosis, with its abundance of dietary fats and oils may actually help your dieting efforts. Understanding more about ketones and their place in a ketogenic diet may assist your food choices and dietary efforts.

In addition to their role in weight loss and weight management, different types of dietary fats and oils and ketones are important for brain function, some disease protection and management, and overall health if used advantageously and correctly.

Dietary fats and oils are naturally found in foods and beverages such as dairy products, eggs, nuts, meats and seeds. Manufactured dietary fats and oils are found in some beverages, processed foods like margarine, cheeses and meats. Ketones are produced by the human body—you'll soon discover how.

There are differing viewpoints on the benefits of different types of dietary fats and oils and about ketones, the ideal amounts to consume and how ketones may sensibly be used for weight loss.

> **The key is to understand the importance of fats in ketogenic diets *and* how to use them to your advantage.**

The purpose of this book is to help educate you about the types of dietary and blood fats and their contribution to health, and their relation to ketones and the ketogenic diet. It provides you with recipes that focus on healthy fats, proteins and non-starchy vegetables and de-emphasizes carbohydrates—particularly those that are refined or processed.

Your healthcare provider may help you determine if these approaches to eating and dieting are appropriate for you, so ask your doctor before you begin this or any other diet program.

Choose the Right Fats

Fats are essential for proper body functioning and contribute satisfaction to diets, plus fats add flavor to foods and beverages. Still, fats provide more than twice the number of calories as carbohydrates or proteins (9 calories per gram compared to 4 calories per gram respectively). On a ketogenic diet, there is a different approach to fats than other diets that may restrict fats. The key is to understand the importance of fats in ketogenic diets and how to use them to your advantage.

Types of Fats

Saturated fats are primarily found in foods from animal sources, such as meat, poultry and full-fat dairy products, while trans fats are mostly created when oils are partially hydrogenated to improve their cooking applications and to give them a longer shelf life. Saturated and trans fats may place a person at greater risk for heart disease. On the other hand, unsaturated fats that include monounsaturated and polyunsaturated fatty acids, found in plant-based foods such as avocados, nuts and seeds and olives and olive oil, and in fatty fish such as salmon, sardines and tuna tend to lower the risk of heart issues.

The American Heart Association (AHA) Diet and Lifestyle Recommendations suggest that a person limit saturated and trans fats and replace them with monounsaturated and polyunsaturated fats. If blood cholesterol needs to be lowered, then the recommendation is to reduce saturated fat to no more than 5 to 6 percent of total calories. For someone consuming 2,000 calories a day, this is about 13 grams of saturated fat, or about 117 calories. This is the equivalent of about 1 ounce of Cheddar cheese (9.4% total fat with 6 grams of saturated fat) and about 3 ounces of regular ground beef (25% total fat with 6.1 grams of saturated fat).

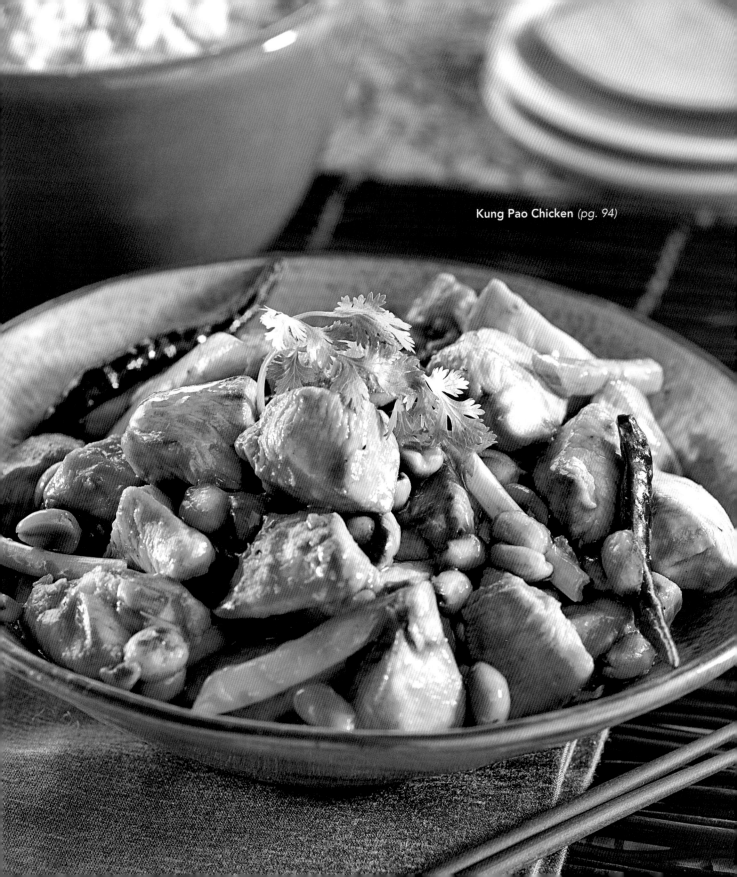

Kung Pao Chicken *(pg. 94)*

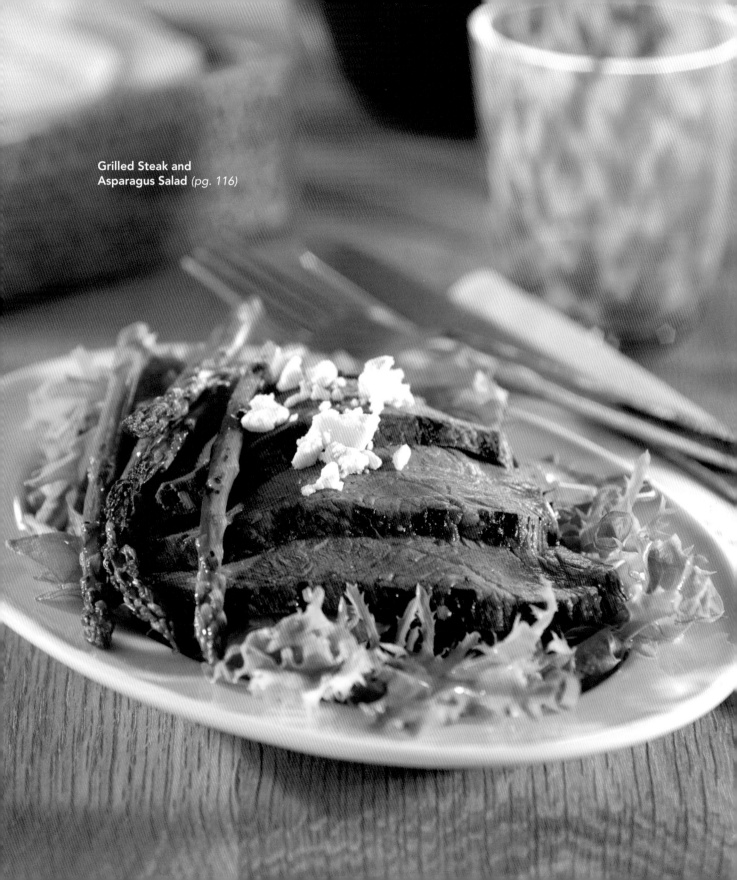

Grilled Steak and
Asparagus Salad *(pg. 116)*

Try to eliminate trans fats (fats that have been processed into saturated fats) completely, or limit them to less than 1 percent of total daily calories. On a 2,000-calorie diet, this means that fewer than 20 calories (about 2 grams) should be derived from trans fats.

The Ketogenic Diet and Dieting

The ketogenic diet is hardly new. The idea that fasting could be used as a therapy to treat disease was one that ancient Greek and Indian physicians embraced. "On the Sacred Disease," an early treatise in the Hippocratic Corpus, proposed how dietary modifications could be useful in epileptic management. Hippocrates, a Greek physician called the Father of Modern Medicine, wrote in "Epidemics" how abstinence from food and drink cured epilepsy.

In the 20th century, the first ketogenic diet became popularized in the 1920's and 30's as a regimen for treating epilepsy and an alternative to non-mainstream fasting. It was also promoted as a means of restoring health. In 1921, the ketogenic diet was officially established when an endocrinologist noted that three water-soluble compounds were produced by the liver as a result of following a diet that was rich in fat and low in carbohydrates. The term "water diet" had been used prior to this time to describe a diet that was free of starch and sugar. This is because when carbohydrates are broken down by the body carbon dioxide and water are by-products. When newer, anticonvulsant therapies were established, the ketogenic diet was temporarily abandoned.

In the 1960's the ketogenic diet was revisited when it was noted that more ketones are produced by medium chain triglycerides (MCTs) per unit of energy than by normal dietary fats (mostly long-chain triglycerides) because MCTs are quickly transported to the liver to be metabolized. In research diets where about 60 percent of the calories came from MCT oil, more protein and up to about three times as many carbohydrates could be consumed in comparison to "classic" ketogenic diets. This is why MCT oil is included in some ketogenic diets today.

In the 1950's and 1960's many versions of the ketogenic diet were popularized as high-protein, low-carbohydrate and a quick method of weight loss. Also at this time, the risk factors of excess fat and protein in the diet were criticized for being detrimental to health. Outside of the medical community, the ketogenic diet was not widely recognized for its therapeutic benefits so response to it was sensational in scope.

TABLE 1

KETOGENIC DIET BASICS

Generally, the percentages of macronutrients on a ketogenic diet are as follows:

- **Fat** 60 to 75 percent of total daily calories
- **Protein** 15 to 30 percent of total daily calories
- **Carbohydrates** 5 to 10 percent of total daily calories

Both fat and protein have high priority on a ketogenic diet, with non-starchy carbohydrates completing the remaining calories. While calories are not as important on the ketogenic diet as they are for other diets, a closer examination of the contributions of these macronutrients helps to put the amounts into perspective.

If total daily calories were about 2,000, then the percentages of macronutrients on a ketogenic diet would resemble the following amounts:

- **Fat** 60 to 75 percent of total daily calories or about 1,200 to 1,500 calories
- **Protein** 15 to 30 percent of total daily calories or about 300 to 600 calories
- **Carbohydrates** 5 to 10 percent of total daily calories or about 100 to 200 calories

In selecting foods and beverages, think protein and fat first, then non-starchy carbohydrates to complete. Until you truly have a handle on what constitutes low carbohydrates, find a carbohydrate counter to help to keep you in line. The ketogenic diet meal suggestions in **Table 5 – SAMPLE KETOGENIC DIET MEALS: BREAKFAST, LUNCH, DINNER AND SNACKS** on page 24 may help your food and beverage selections.

Then in the 1980's the Glycemic Index (GI) of foods and beverages was revealed that accounted for the differences in the speed of digestion of different types of carbohydrates. This explanation became the springboard for a number of ketogenic diets that were revised from years earlier. By the late 1990's the low-carb craze became one of the most popular types of dieting. Since this time, the original ketogenic diet underwent many refinements and hybrid diets developed.

Variations of the ketogenic diet continued to surface throughout the 20th century since the premise of the ketogenic diet—higher fat and protein and low carbohydrate—was used to treat diabetes and induce weight loss among other applications.

Table 1 summarizes the ketogenic diet basics. Many clinical studies examined their effectiveness and safety and their advantages and drawbacks were identified. These are condensed in Table 2.

TABLE 2

ADVANTAGES AND DRAWBACKS OF KETOGENIC DIETS

ADVANTAGES

- No calorie counting or focus on portion sizes
- Initial weight loss
- After initial transition, hunger subsides
- Improved energy
- Improved blood pressure
- Improved blood fats: high-density lipoproteins, cholesterol, low-density lipoproteins, triglycerides
- Reduced blood sugar, C-reactive protein (marker of inflammation), insulin, waist circumference
- Significant short-term weight loss possible

DRAWBACKS

- Hard to sustain
- Limited food choices
- May lead to taste fatigue
- Socialization difficult
- Digestive issues (such as constipation, fatty stool, nausea)
- Nutrient deficiencies (such as calcium, vitamins A, C and D, B-vitamins, fiber, magnesium, selenium)
- Fiber, vitamin and mineral supplements suggested
- Increased urination (bladder, kidney contraindications)
- Diabetes issues
- Rapid, sizeable short-term weight loss concerning; long-term weight maintenance questionable

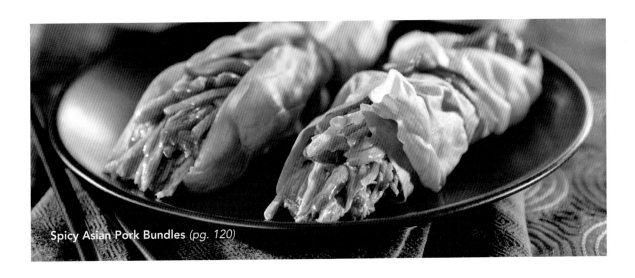

Spicy Asian Pork Bundles *(pg. 120)*

One of the most important roles of fat in the body is as an energy source, especially when carbohydrates are not available from the diet or are lacking in the body.

Fat in Health and Disease

Fats are essential to the diet and health for many purposes. Fats function as the body's thermostat. The layer of fat just beneath the skin helps to keep the body warm or causes it to perspire to cool the body.

Fat contributes to bile acids, cell membranes and steroid hormones (such as estrogen and testosterone), cushions the body from shock and helps to regulate fluid balance. Too many or too few fats in the diet may influence each of these important body functions.

One of the most important roles of fat in the body is as an energy source, especially when carbohydrates are not available from the diet or are lacking in the body. When people did manual work all day and expended the calories that they consumed, they made good use of carbohydrates and fats in their diet and within their energy stores. Today's laborsaving devices and sedentary lifestyles create less need for excess carbohydrate calories—particularly if they are refined. Even a plant-based diet may be unnecessarily high in refined carbohydrate calories.

Over the years, as humans moved from a plant-based diet toward an animal-based diet, the composition of fatty acids in the American diet switched from monounsaturated and polyunsaturated fats to more saturated fats, which are associated more with cardiovascular disease. A diet that is only filled with saturated fats may not be healthy. Incorporating avocado, fish, nuts, oils and seeds and other foods that contain monounsaturated and polyunsaturated fats into your diet may help to support a healthier proportion of fats in the body for weight maintenance and good health.

Besides cardiovascular disease, excess saturated and trans fats in the human diet are associated with certain cancers, cerebral vascular disease, diabetes, obesity and metabolic syndrome (a collection of conditions that may include abnormal cholesterol or triglyceride levels, excess body fat around the waist, high blood sugar and increased blood pressure that may increase a person's risk of diabetes, heart disease and/or stroke).

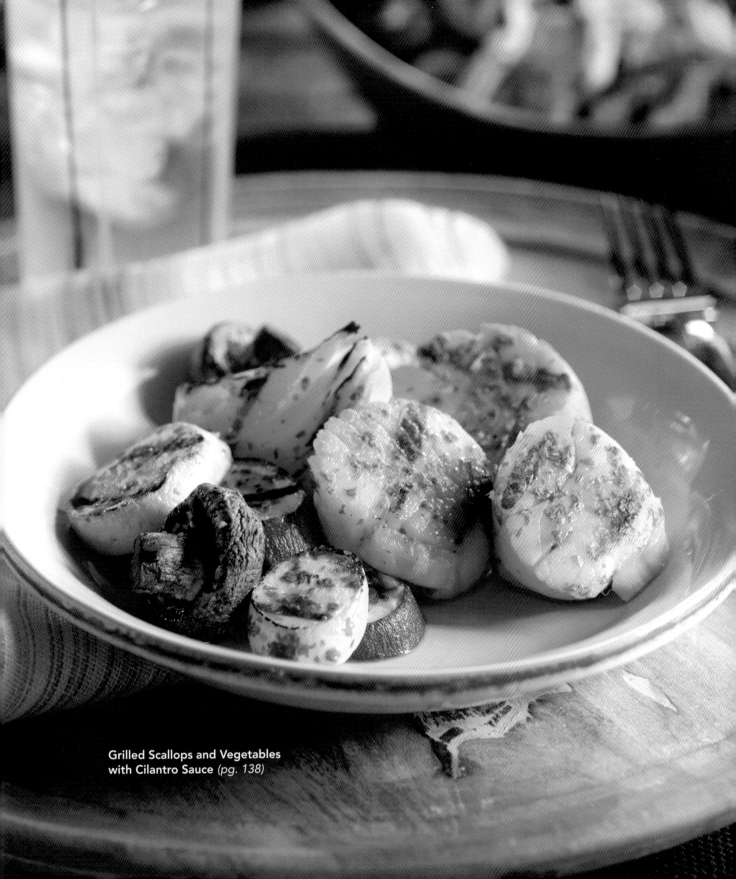

Grilled Scallops and Vegetables
with Cilantro Sauce *(pg. 138)*

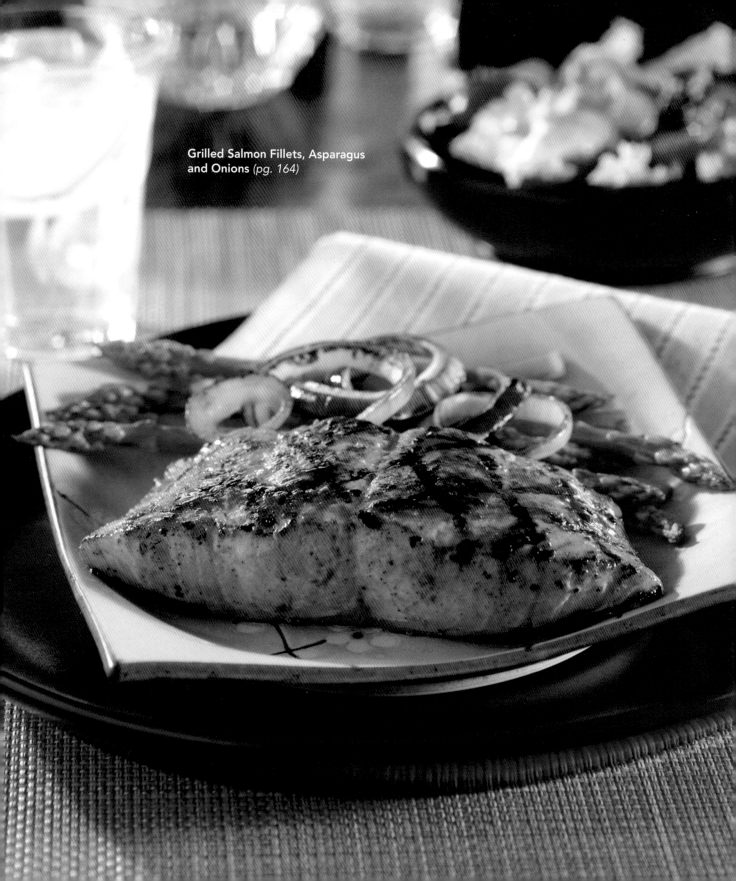

Grilled Salmon Fillets, Asparagus and Onions *(pg. 164)*

The Cholesterol Controversy

Atherosclerosis, or hardening of the arteries, is not a modern disease. Rather, the association between blood cholesterol and cardiovascular disease was recognized as far back as the 1850's.

One hundred years later in the 1950's, cholesterol and saturated fats in the diet were implicated as major risk factors for cardiovascular disease. Then in the 1980's, major US health institutions established that the process of lowering blood cholesterol (specifically LDL-cholesterol) reduces the risk of heart attacks that are caused by coronary heart disease.

Some scientists questioned this conclusion that marked the unofficial start of what's been called the "cholesterol controversy." Studies of cholesterol-lowering drugs known as statins supported the idea that reducing blood cholesterol means less mortality from heart disease. Subsequent statin studies have questioned this association. Other factors aside from dietary cholesterol have since been identified that may lead to elevated blood cholesterol, such as trans fats.

The liver manufactures cholesterol, so reducing cholesterol in the diet should help to reduce blood cholesterol, coronary heart disease and the risk of heart attack. But in some individuals, the liver produces more cholesterol than the body requires and cardiovascular disease may still develop. Accordingly, dietary cholesterol does not necessarily predict cardiovascular disease or a heart attack.

While dietary cholesterol may be a measure for greater cardiovascular risks, cardiovascular disease and heart attacks are also dependent upon such lifestyle and genetic factors as age, diet, exercise, gender, genetics, medication and stress. Reducing hydrogenated fats, saturated fats and trans fats; incorporating mono- and polyunsaturated fats and losing weight to help better manage blood fats are other sensible measures to take.

Longer-term weight management is also a preventative measure in cardiovascular disease. Reducing cholesterol and saturated fat in the diet while integrating foods and beverages with mono- and polyunsaturated fats and oils, dietary fiber, antioxidants and other phytonutrients may lead to a decrease in overall calorie consumption and weight loss and an improvement in overall health.

So What (and How) Should I Eat?

If you want to lose body fat, then the general consensus is that you need to take in fewer calories than you burn for energy. For example, if you're an average woman over 40, decreasing your caloric intake may be a reasonable starting point. If you are of shorter stature and/or very inactive, or you haven't dropped any pounds after a few weeks, you may consider lowering your daily intake of calories by 100-calorie increments until you start seeing weight loss. But don't go much below 1,000 calories without your health care provider's supervision. (And be sure to check with your health care provider before making any major changes to your diet or activity level, especially if you have any serious health problems.)

Another approach to weight loss is the ketogenic diet that does not focus on calories. Instead, the ketogenic diet focuses on the composition of calories from fats, proteins and carbohydrates.

Fats are satisfying because they take longer for the body to digest, and some are converted into ketones for energy. You don't want to skimp on proteins because protein helps maintain and build calorie-burning muscle and also keeps you satiated between meals. Choose protein sources that supply monounsaturated fats and other heart-healthy unsaturated fats; good options include fish, seafood, nuts and seeds. (Fatty fish, such as herring, mackerel, salmon and tuna contain polyunsaturated fats—especially disease-fighting omega-3 fatty acids). You'll need to replace highly processed and refined foods that are full of saturated and trans fats, sugar and refined carbohydrates with minimally processed fiber- and nutrient-rich foods that include non-starchy vegetables.

What you'll likely end up with is a satisfying eating plan with ample protein, healthy fats and minimal carbohydrates that may help you to feel full and lose weight in the process. It's also a plan that may help you to maintain weight loss over time in a modified manner.

If you've ever tried to lose weight before, you know how quickly between-meal hunger may sabotage your best efforts. When your stomach starts rumbling hours before your next meal, it's tempting to grab whatever is available. Often, that "whatever" is some unhealthy packaged snack food or beverage that is loaded with empty calories, sodium, sugars and/or unhealthy fats. Or, if you manage to ignore this hunger, you may become so ravenous at the next meal that you consume far more calories than your body actually needs.

Bacon-Tomato Grilled Cheese *(pg. 186)*

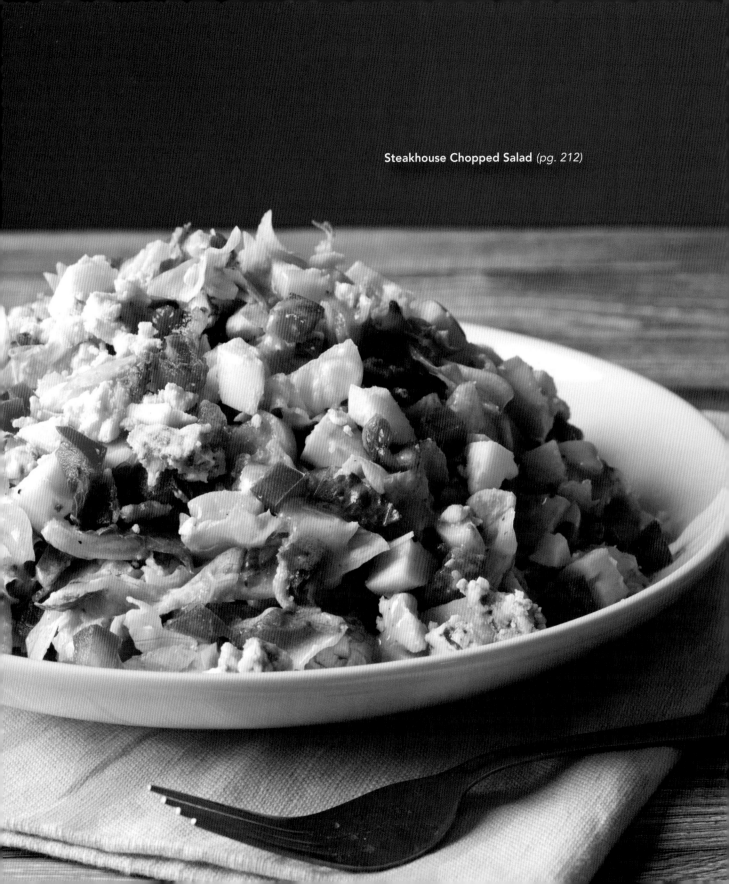

Steakhouse Chopped Salad *(pg. 212)*

> What you'll likely end up with is a satisfying eating plan with ample protein, healthy fats *and* minimal carbohydrates that may help you to feel full *and* lose weight in the process.

To prevent hunger from spoiling your weight-loss efforts, eat when you are hungry and stop eating when you are full, whether a meal or snack. Try to consume meals and snacks that include a source of hunger-fighting protein and healthy fat, and count your carbs so as not to exceed the daily limit of 20 to 50 grams of non-starchy carbohydrates.

Drink plenty of water throughout the day (especially if you live in a hot climate or sweat excessively) since ketogenic diets tend to be dehydrating and may lead to fatigue or ill feelings. This may be due to an imbalance of electrolytes; specifically sodium that the kidneys excrete during ketosis. Sometimes lightly salting your food may help to restore sodium. A high-quality vitamin and mineral supplement is also sensible.

Notes on Ketogenic Foods, Beverages and Ingredients

In general, the foods, beverages and ingredients that are included in a ketogenic diet incorporate eggs, healthy fats and oils, fish, meats and organ meats and non-starchy vegetables. These "acceptable" foods, beverages and ingredients contain protein and fats and are low in carbohydrates that contribute to the effectiveness of ketogenic diets. They are listed in Table 3 – ACCEPTABLE FOODS, BEVERAGES AND INGREDIENTS FOR KETOGENIC DIETS.

In Table 4 – UNACCEPTABLE FOODS, BEVERAGES AND INGREDIENTS FOR KETOGENIC DIETS are shown. While there is a wide-range of ketogenic diet approaches, these foods, beverages and ingredients are generally considered to be "unacceptable" on many ketogenic diets. In general, their carbohydrate content exceeds what is considered as optimal for effective ketosis and diet success.

TABLE 3

ACCEPTABLE FOODS, BEVERAGES AND INGREDIENTS FOR KETOGENIC DIETS

BEVERAGES

- Broth
- Hard liquor
- Nut milks
- Unsweetened coffee, tea
- Water

EGGS

- Egg whites
- Powdered eggs
- Whole eggs

FATS AND OILS

- Butter
- Cocoa butter
- Coconut butter, cream and oil
- Ghee
- Lard
- Oils: avocado oil, macadamia nut oil, MCT oil, olive oil and cold-pressed vegetable oils (flax, safflower, soybean)
- Mayonnaise

FISH AND SEAFOOD

- Anchovies
- Fish (catfish, cod, flounder, halibut, mackerel, mahi-mahi, salmon, snapper, trout, tuna)
- Shellfish (clams, crab, lobster, mussels, oysters, scallops, squid)

FRUITS AND VEGETABLES

- Avocados
- Cruciferous vegetables (broccoli, brussels sprouts, cabbage, cauliflower, kohlrabi)
- Fermented vegetables (kimchi, sauerkraut)
- Leafy greens (bok choy, chard, endive, lettuce, kale, radicchio, spinach, watercress)
- Lemon and lime juice and peel
- Mushrooms
- Non-starchy vegetables (asparagus, bamboo shoots, celery, cucumber)
- Seaweed and kelp
- Squash (spaghetti squash, yellow squash, zucchini)
- Tomatoes (used in moderation in some keto diets)

DAIRY PRODUCTS

- Crème fraîche
- Greek yogurt
- Hard cheese (aged Cheddar, feta, Parmesan, Swiss)
- Heavy cream
- Soft cheese (Brie, blue, Colby, Monterey Jack, mozzarella)
- Sour cream
- Spreadable cheese (cream cheese, cottage cheese and mascarpone)

MEATS AND POULTRY

- Beef (ground beef, roasts, steak, stew meat)
- Goat (leg, loin, rack, saddle, shoulder)
- Lamb (leg, loin, rack, ribs, shank, shoulder)
- Organ meats (heart, kidneys, liver, tongue)
- Poultry with skin (such as chicken, duck, pheasant, quail, turkey)
- Pork (bacon and sausage without fillers, ground pork, ham, pork chops, pork loin, tenderloin)
- Tofu used in moderation in some keto diets)
- Veal (double, flank, leg, rib, shoulder, sirloin)

NON-DAIRY BEVERAGES

- Almond milk
- Cashew milk
- Coconut milk
- Soymilk (used in moderation in some keto diets)

NUTS AND SEEDS

- Nut butters (almond, macadamia)
- Seeds (chia, flax, poppy, sesame, sunflower)
- Whole nuts (almonds, Brazil nuts, macadamia, pecans, hazelnuts, pine nuts, walnuts)

PANTRY ITEMS

- Herbs (dried or fresh such as basil, cilantro, oregano, parsley, rosemary and thyme)
- Horseradish
- Hot sauce
- Mustard
- Pepper
- Pesto sauce
- Pickles
- Salad dressings (without sweeteners)
- Salt
- Spices (such as ground red pepper, chili powder, cinnamon and cumin)
- Unsweetened gelatin
- Vinegar
- Whey protein (unsweetened)
- Worcestershire sauce

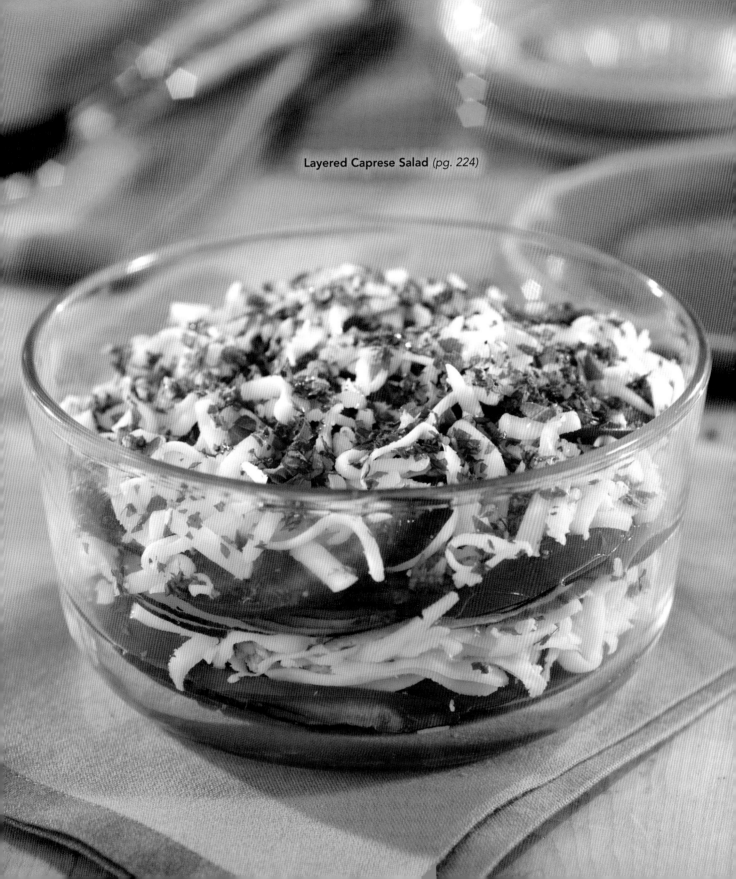

Layered Caprese Salad (pg. 224)

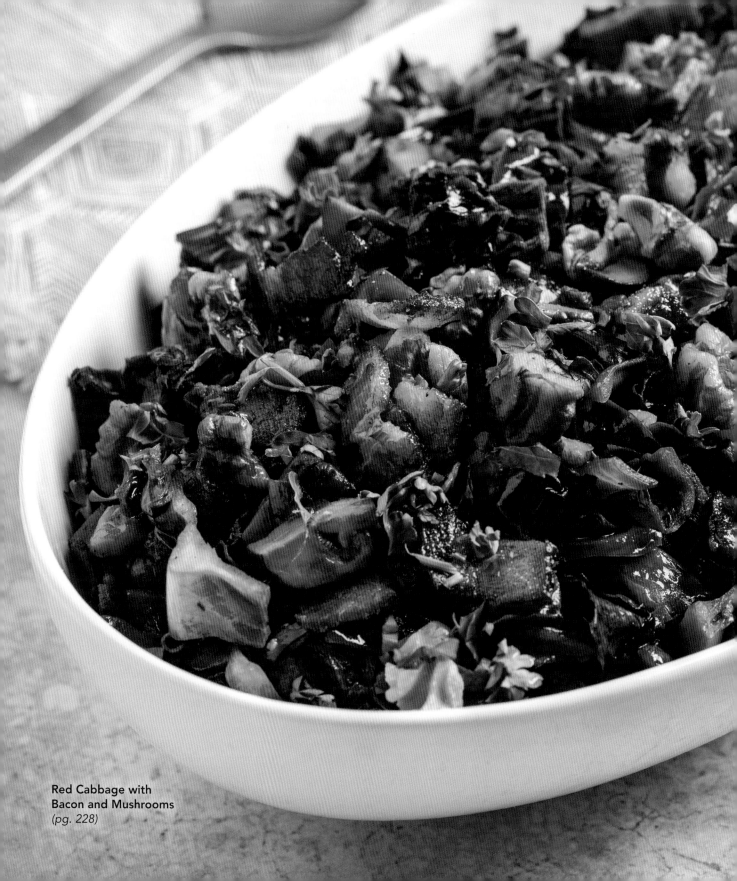

Red Cabbage with
Bacon and Mushrooms
(pg. 228)

TABLE 4

UNACCEPTABLE FOODS, BEVERAGES AND INGREDIENTS FOR KETOGENIC DIETS

- Alcohol other than hard liquor (beer, sugary alcoholic beverages, wine)
- Beans
- Breads and breadstuffs
- Cakes and pastries
- Candy
- Cereals
- Cookies
- Crackers
- Flours
- Fruit, all (fresh, dried)
- Grains (amaranth, barley, buckwheat, bulgur, corn, millet, oats, rice, rye, sorghum, sprouted grains, wheat)
- Legumes (lentils, peas)
- Margarines with trans fats
- Milk (full-fat milk is acceptable in some ketogenic diets)
- Oats and muesli
- Potatoes, all kinds (white, yellow, sweet)
- Quinoa
- Pasta
- Pizza
- Processed and refined snack foods
- Rice
- Root vegetables
- Soda
- Sports drinks
- Sugar and honey
- Syrup
- Wheat gluten
- Yams

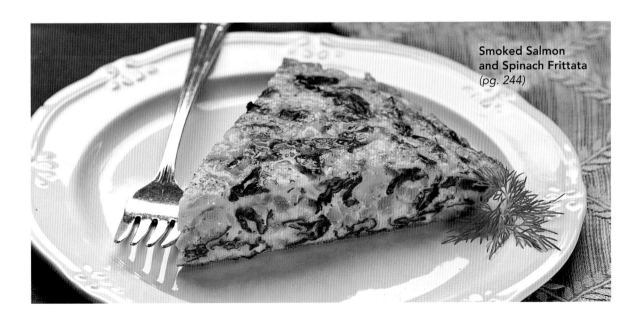

Smoked Salmon and Spinach Frittata (*pg. 244*)

TABLE 5

SAMPLE KETOGENIC DIET MEALS: BREAKFAST, LUNCH, DINNER AND SNACKS

Examples of combinations of protein, low-carb, non-starchy vegetables and fats:

BREAKFAST:

- Almond, coconut, hemp or other nut or seed milks or beverages (unsweetened)
- Bacon, sausage or sliced meats (without carbohydrate fillers)
- Cheese, hard or soft varieties
- Eggs, scrambled or fried + vegetables (asparagus, broccoli, garlic, mushrooms, onions or spinach) + coconut or olive oil + avocado, olives, salsa and/or sour cream
- Greek yogurt with nut butter, chia or flax seeds, herbs and spices (cinnamon, ginger or nutmeg)
- Smoked fish (such as lox, sable or whitefish)
- Smoothies made with keto-friendly ingredients (protein powder, almond or coconut butter, avocado, cocoa powder, chia or flax seeds, spices such as cinnamon, smoked paprika or turmeric and unsweetened almond or hemp milk)
- Vegetable slices (cucumber or zucchini or lettuce) topped with cheese

LUNCH AND DINNER:

- Eggs + watercress or spinach + avocado dressing
- Lamb + kale + sesame oil
- Pork + cauliflower + coconut butter
- Poultry + zucchini and yellow squash + extra virgin olive oil
- Salmon + broccoli + mustard sauce
- Sardines + cucumbers and onions + sour cream dressing
- Seafood + leafy green salad + oil and vinegar dressing
- Steak + asparagus + butter sauce
- Tofu + mushrooms and bok choy + ghee
- Tuna + celery + mayonnaise

SNACKS:

- Asparagus with goat cheese dip
- Avocado filled hard-cooked eggs
- Celery + nut or seed butter
- Cheese + olive skewers
- Chia and flaxseed crackers + cream cheese
- Cucumber and cream cheese spread
- Cream cheese and bacon stuffed celery
- Deviled eggs with fresh herbs and chives
- Greek yogurt with chopped cucumbers and garlic
- Guacamole with onions and garlic
- Ham and Cheddar or Swiss cheese roll ups
- Mixed nut-coated cheese balls
- Nut butters (such as almond) blended with ricotta cheese
- Olives stuffed with blue cheese
- Parmesan cheese crisps
- Seeds and seed butters such as tahini
- Sliced jicama with herbed cream cheese

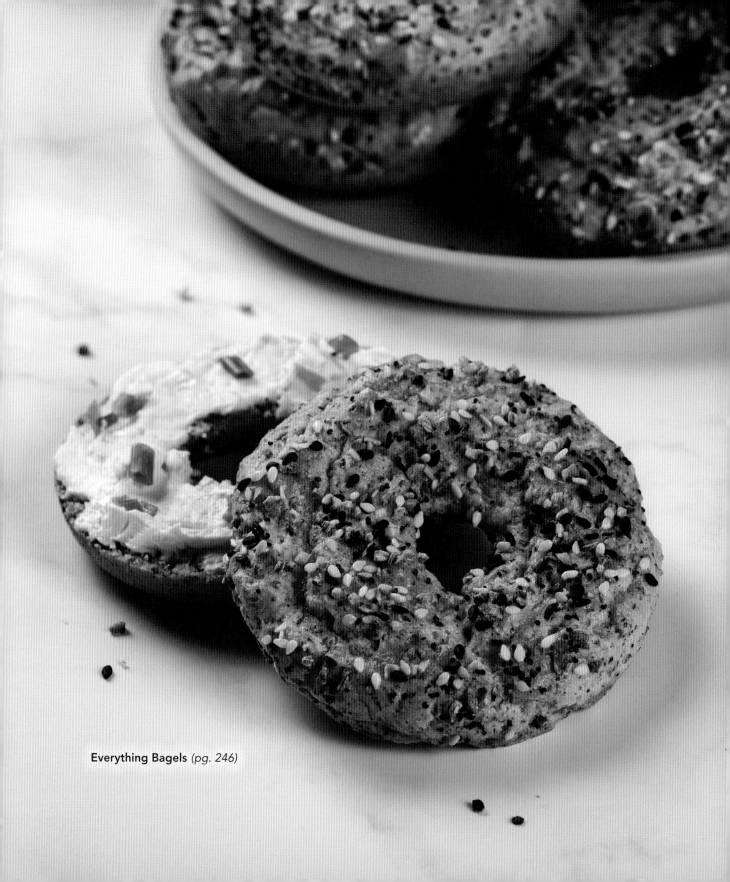

Everything Bagels *(pg. 246)*

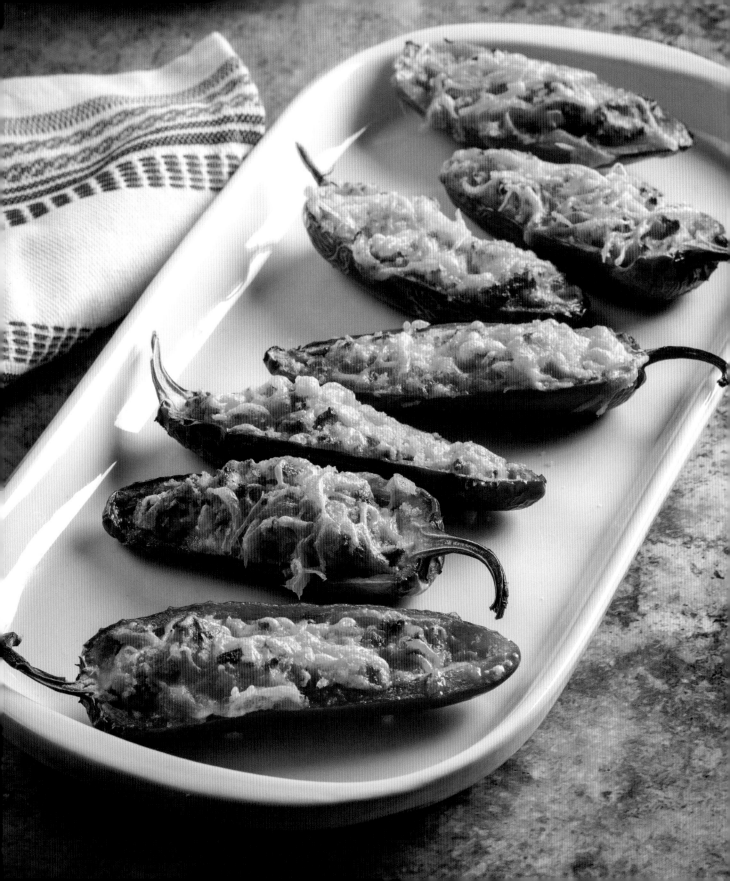

snacks *and* appetizers

PER SERVING

110 calories
10g **total fat**
2g **carbs**
2g **net carbs**
0g **dietary fiber**
4g **protein**

Jalapeño Poppers

makes 20 to 24 poppers

10 to 12 fresh jalapeño peppers*

1 package (8 ounces) cream cheese, softened

1½ cups (6 ounces) shredded Cheddar cheese, divided

2 green onions, finely chopped

½ teaspoon onion powder

¼ teaspoon salt

⅛ teaspoon garlic powder

6 slices bacon, crisp cooked and finely chopped

2 tablespoons almond flour (optional)

2 tablespoons grated Parmesan or Romano cheese

For large jalapeño peppers, use 10. For small peppers, use 12.

1. Preheat oven to 375°F. Line baking sheet with parchment paper or foil.

2. Cut each pepper in half lengthwise; remove ribs and seeds.

3. Combine cream cheese, 1 cup Cheddar cheese, green onions, onion powder, salt and garlic powder in medium bowl. Stir in bacon. Fill each pepper half with about 1 tablespoon cheese mixture. Place on prepared baking sheet. Sprinkle with remaining ½ cup Cheddar cheese, almond flour, if desired, and Parmesan cheese.

4. Bake 10 to 12 minutes or until cheese is melted but peppers are still firm.

Eggplant Rolls

makes 6 servings (2 rolls per serving)

1 large eggplant (about 1¼ pounds)

3 tablespoons extra virgin olive oil

Salt and black pepper

1 cup ricotta cheese

½ cup grated Asiago cheese

¼ cup julienned or chopped oil-packed sun-dried tomatoes

¼ cup chopped fresh basil or Italian parsley

⅛ teaspoon red pepper flakes

1. Preheat broiler. Trim stem end from eggplant; discard. Peel eggplant, if desired. Cut eggplant lengthwise into 6 slices about ¼ inch thick. Brush both sides of eggplant slices with oil; season with salt. Place on rack of broiler pan.

2. Broil 4 inches from heat 4 to 5 minutes per side or until golden brown and slightly softened. Let cool to room temperature.

3. Combine ricotta cheese, Asiago cheese, sun-dried tomatoes, basil and red pepper flakes in small bowl; mix well. Season with salt and black pepper to taste.

4. Spread ricotta mixture evenly over eggplant slices. Roll up and cut each roll in half crosswise. Arrange rolls, seam side down, on serving platter. Serve warm or at room temperature.

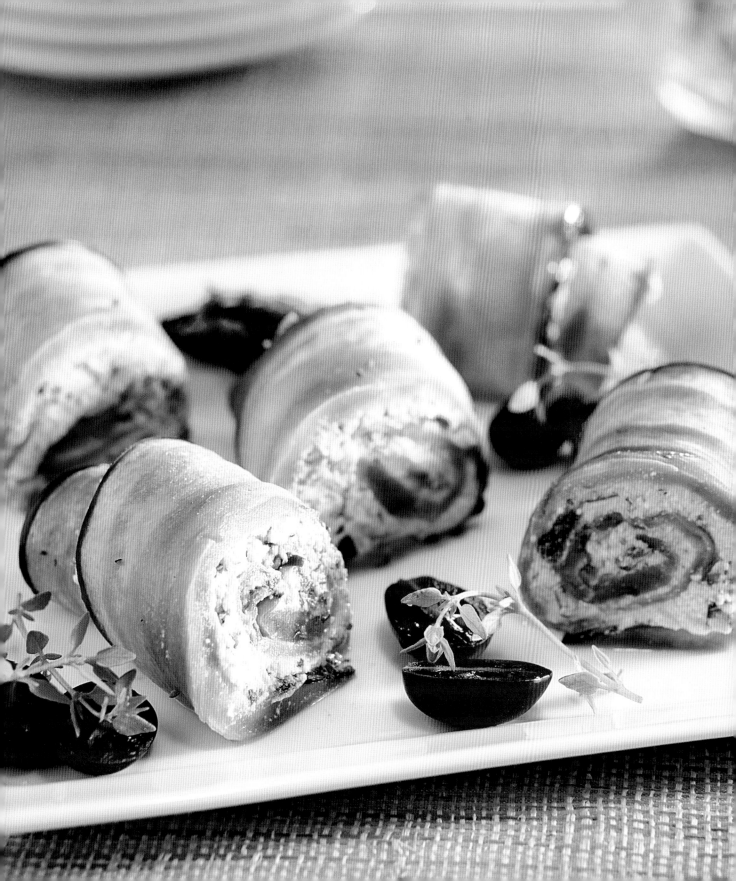

Mushrooms Rockefeller

makes 18 appetizers

PER SERVING

25 calories
1g **total fat**
2g **carbs**
1g **net carbs**
1g **dietary fiber**
2g **protein**

18 large button mushrooms
    (about 1 pound)

 2 slices bacon

¼ cup chopped onion

 1 package (10 ounces) frozen
    chopped spinach, thawed
    and squeezed dry

 1 jar (2 ounces) chopped
    pimientos, drained

 1 tablespoon lemon juice

 1 teaspoon grated lemon peel

1. Spray 13×9-inch baking dish with nonstick cooking spray. Preheat oven to 375°F. Wipe mushrooms clean with damp paper towel. Pull stem out of each mushroom cap.

2. Cut thin slice from base of each stem; discard. Chop stems.

3. Cook bacon in medium skillet over medium heat until crisp. Transfer bacon to paper towels to drain. Add mushroom stems and onion to hot drippings in skillet; cook and stir until onion is tender. Add spinach, pimientos, lemon juice and lemon peel; mix well.

4. Stuff mushroom caps with spinach mixture; place in single layer in prepared baking dish. Crumble bacon; sprinkle over tops of mushrooms. Bake 15 minutes or until heated through. Serve immediately.

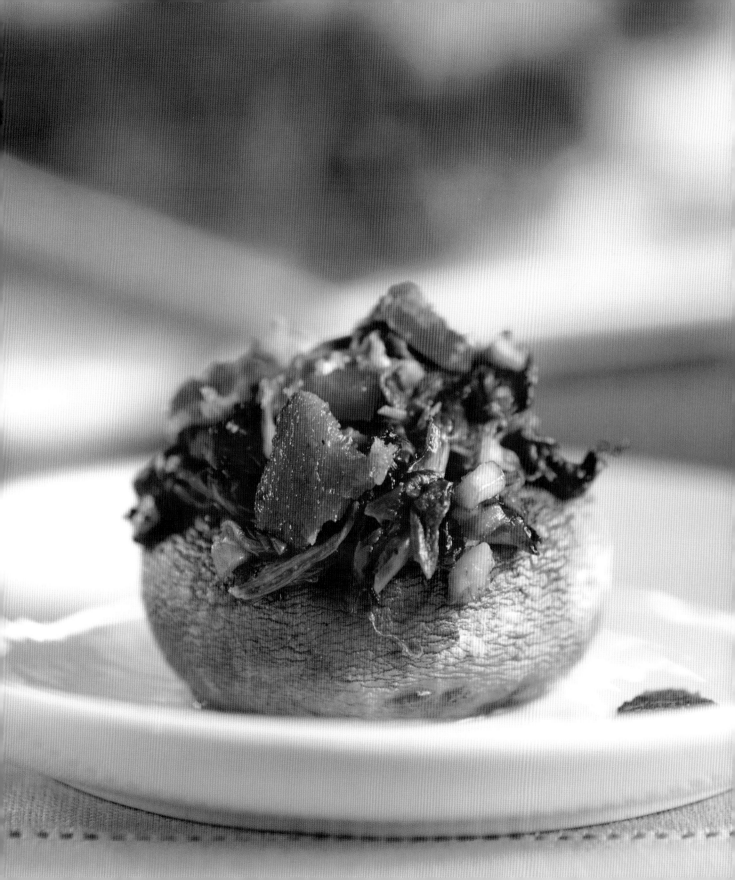

Chorizo and Caramelized Onion Tortilla

makes 36 pieces

2 tablespoons olive oil

3 medium yellow onions, thinly sliced

½ pound Spanish chorizo (about 2 links) or andouille sausage, diced

6 eggs

Salt and black pepper

½ cup chopped fresh parsley

1. Heat oil in medium skillet over medium heat. Add onions; cover and cook 10 minutes or until onions are translucent. Reduce heat to low; cook, uncovered, 40 minutes or until golden and very tender. Transfer onions to bowl.

2. Cook chorizo in same skillet over medium heat 5 minutes or just until chorizo begins to brown, stirring occasionally. Remove from heat; set aside to cool.

3. Preheat oven to 350°F. Spray 9-inch square baking pan with olive oil cooking spray.

4. Whisk eggs in medium bowl; season with salt and pepper. Add onions, chorizo and parsley; stir gently until well blended. Pour egg mixture into prepared pan.

5. Bake 12 to 15 minutes or until center is almost set. *Turn oven to broil.* Broil 1 to 2 minutes or until top just starts to brown. Transfer pan to wire rack; cool completely. Cut into 36 triangles or squares; serve cold or at room temperature.

Tip: The tortilla can be made up to 1 day ahead and refrigerated until serving. To serve at room temperature, remove from refrigerator 30 minutes before serving.

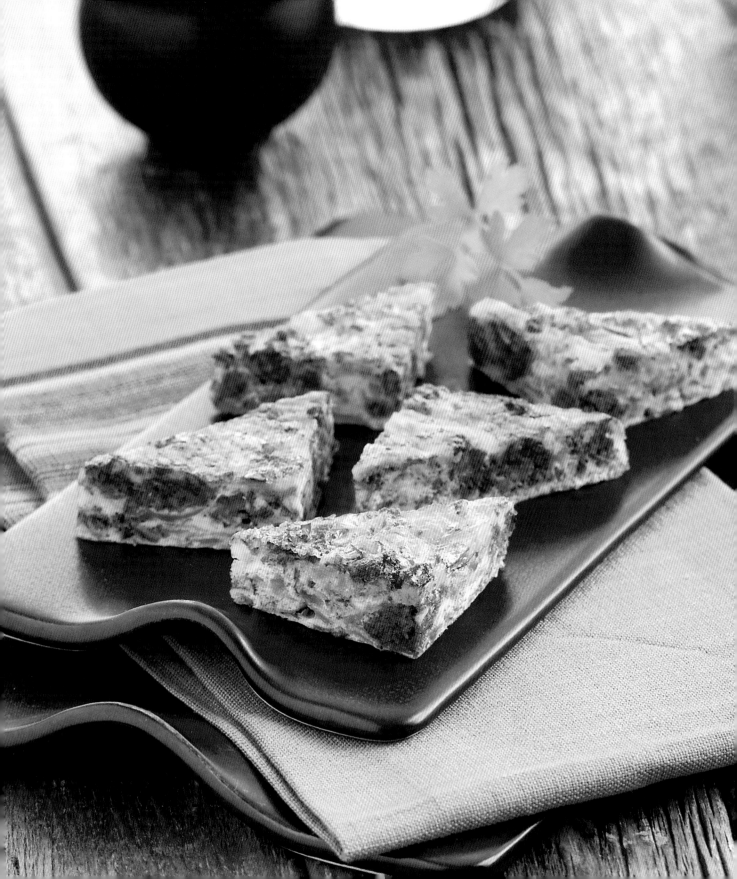

Quick and Easy Stuffed Mushrooms

makes 8 servings

PER SERVING

50 calories
4g **total fat**
4g **carbs**
3g **net carbs**
1g **dietary fiber**
2g **protein**

16 large mushrooms

½ cup sliced celery

½ cup sliced onion

1 clove garlic

½ cup almond flour

1 teaspoon Worcestershire sauce

½ teaspoon dried marjoram or thyme

⅛ teaspoon ground red pepper
    Dash paprika

1. Remove stems from mushrooms; reserve caps. Place mushroom stems, celery, onion and garlic in food processor; pulse until vegetables are finely chopped.

2. Spray large skillet with nonstick cooking spray. Add vegetable mixture; cook and stir over medium heat 5 minutes or until onion is tender. Remove to bowl. Stir in almond flour, Worcestershire sauce, marjoram and red pepper.

3. Fill mushroom caps evenly with mixture, pressing down firmly. Place about ½ inch apart in shallow baking pan. Spray tops with nonstick cooking spray. Sprinkle with paprika.

4. Preheat oven to 350°F. Bake 15 minutes or until heated through.

Note: Mushrooms can be stuffed up to 1 day ahead. Refrigerate filled mushroom caps, covered, until ready to serve. Bake in preheated 300°F oven 20 minutes or until heated through.

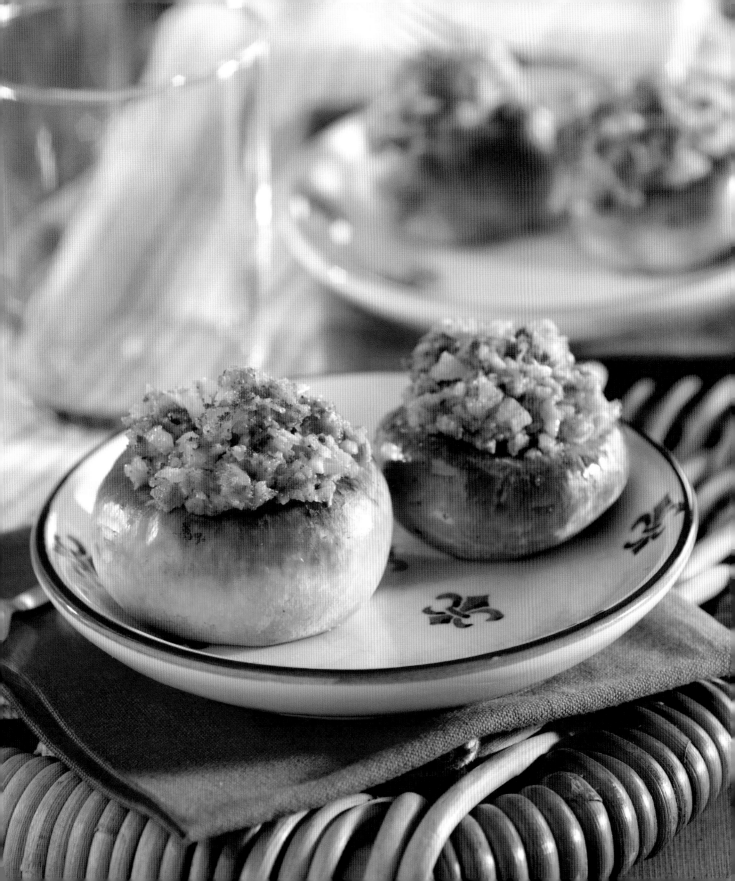

Mini Spinach and Bacon Quiches

makes 12 servings

PER SERVING

180 calories
12g **total fat**
4g **carbs**
3g **net carbs**
1g **dietary fiber**
16g **protein**

3 slices bacon

½ small onion, diced

1 package (10 ounces) frozen chopped spinach, thawed and squeezed dry

½ teaspoon black pepper

⅛ teaspoon ground nutmeg
   Pinch salt

3 eggs

1 container (15 ounces) whole-milk ricotta cheese

2 cups (8 ounces) shredded mozzarella cheese

1 cup grated Parmesan cheese

1. Preheat oven to 350°F. Spray 12 standard (2½-inch) muffin cups with nonstick cooking spray.

2. Cook bacon in large skillet until crisp. Drain on paper towels. Crumble when cool enough to handle.

3. Heat same skillet with bacon drippings over medium heat. Add onion; cook and stir 5 minutes or until tender. Add spinach, pepper, nutmeg and salt; cook and stir 3 minutes or until liquid is evaporated. Remove from heat. Stir in bacon; set aside to cool.

4. Whisk eggs in large bowl. Add cheeses; stir until well blended. Add cooled spinach mixture; mix well. Spoon evenly into prepared muffin cups.

5. Bake 40 minutes or until set. Cool in pan 10 minutes. Run thin knife around edges to remove from pan. Serve immediately.

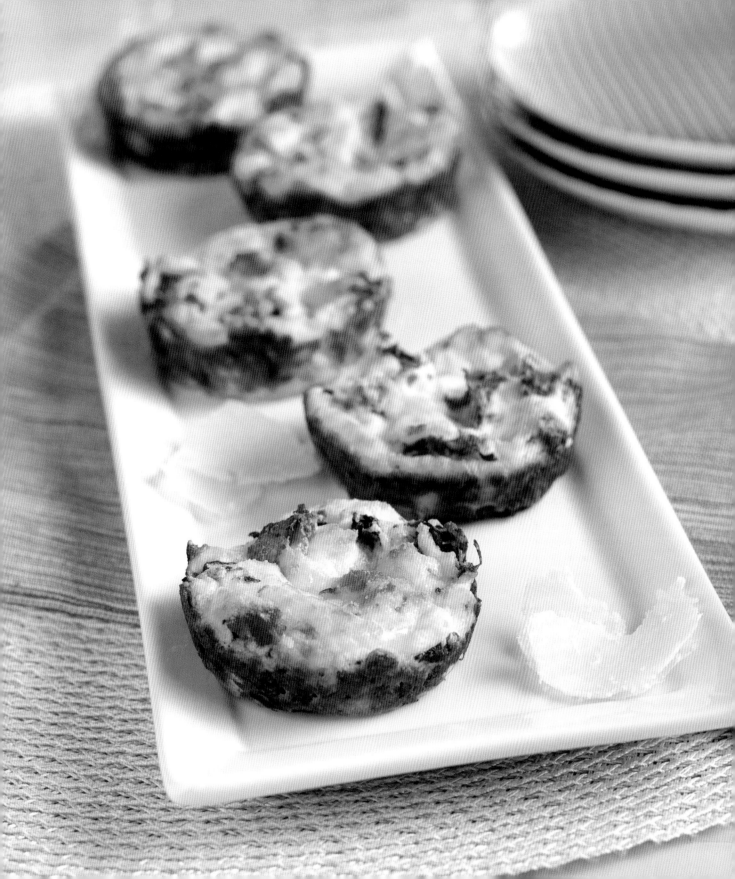

Greek-Style Chicken Wings with Tzatziki Sauce

makes 8 servings

Chicken Wings

- 5 pounds chicken wings, tips removed and split at joints
- 2 tablespoons olive oil, divided
- 2 teaspoons dried oregano
- ½ teaspoon salt
- ¼ teaspoon black pepper
- 2 tablespoons fresh lemon juice

Tzatziki Sauce

- 1 medium cucumber, peeled, halved lengthwise and seeded
- 2 cups plain Greek yogurt
- 2 tablespoons fresh lemon juice
- 2 tablespoons olive oil
- 1 clove garlic, crushed
- ½ teaspoon salt

1. Preheat oven to 375°F.

2. Combine chicken, oil, oregano, ½ teaspoon salt and pepper in large bowl; toss to coat. Spread in single layer on 1 or 2 baking sheets. Bake 1 hour or until crispy and cooked through.

3. Meanwhile for tzatziki sauce, grate cucumber on large holes of box grater into medium bowl. Stir in yogurt, 2 tablespoons lemon juice, 2 tablespoons oil, crushed garlic and ½ teaspoon salt. Cover and refrigerate until ready to serve.

4. Drizzle lemon juice over chicken; stir to coat. Serve with tzatziki sauce.

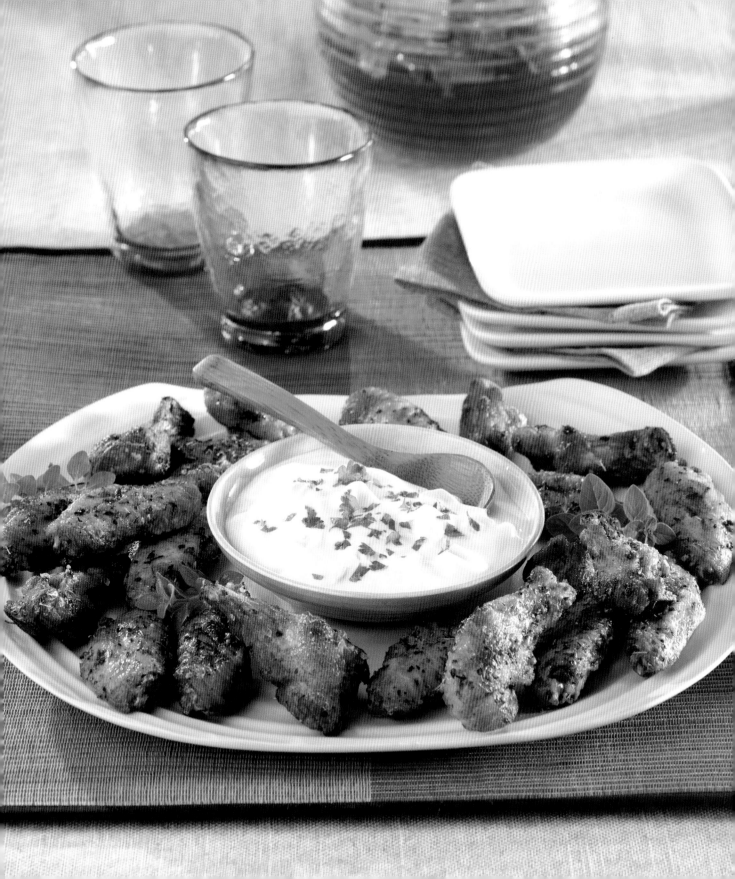

Crab-Stuffed Tomatoes

makes 8 to 10 servings

PER SERVING

70 calories
5g total fat
2g carbs
1g net carbs
1g dietary fiber
4g protein

16 large cherry tomatoes
(1½ inches in diameter)

3 tablespoons mayonnaise

½ teaspoon lemon juice

1 small clove garlic, minced

¾ cup fresh or refrigerated
canned crabmeat*

3 tablespoons chopped pimiento-
stuffed green olives

2 tablespoons slivered almonds
or pine nuts

⅛ teaspoon black pepper

*Choose special grade crabmeat
for this recipe. It is less expensive
and already flaked but just as
flavorful as backfin, lump or
claw meat. Look for it in the
refrigerated seafood section of the
supermarket. Shelf-stable canned
crabmeat can be substituted.*

1. Cut small slivers from bottoms of cherry tomatoes so they will stand upright. Cut off top of tomatoes; scoop out seeds and membranes. Turn tomatoes upside down to drain; set aside.

2. Combine mayonnaise, lemon juice and garlic in medium bowl. Add crabmeat, olives, almonds and pepper; stir gently to coat.

3. Spoon crab mixture into tomatoes. Serve immediately.

Tip: For the best flavor, do not refrigerate the stuffed tomatoes. Crab mixture can be prepared several hours in advance and refrigerated. Stuff tomatoes with the crab mixture just before serving. Or the crab mixture can be served on crackers or toasted French bread rounds.

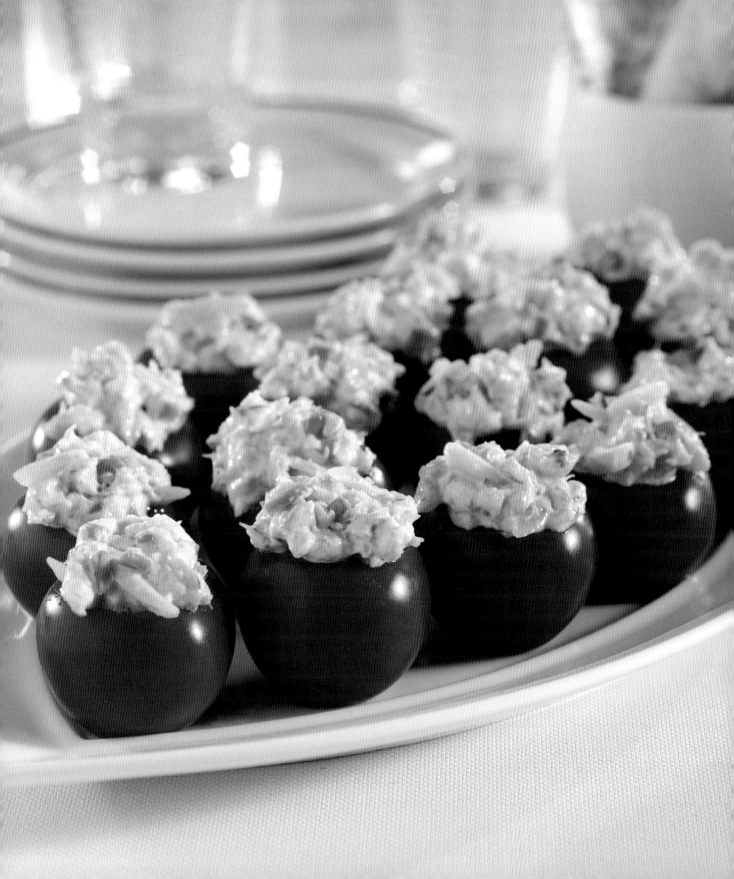

Bell Pepper Wedges with Herbed Goat Cheese

makes 6 servings (2 pieces per serving)

2 small red bell peppers

1 log (4 ounces) plain goat cheese, softened

⅓ cup whipped cream cheese

2 tablespoons minced fresh chives

1 teaspoon minced fresh dill

Fresh dill sprigs (optional)

1. Cut tops off of bell peppers; remove core and seeds. Cut each pepper into 6 wedges. Remove ribs, if necessary.

2. Combine goat cheese, cream cheese, chives and minced dill in small bowl; stir until well blended. Pipe or spread 1 tablespoon goat cheese mixture onto each pepper wedge. Garnish with dill sprigs.

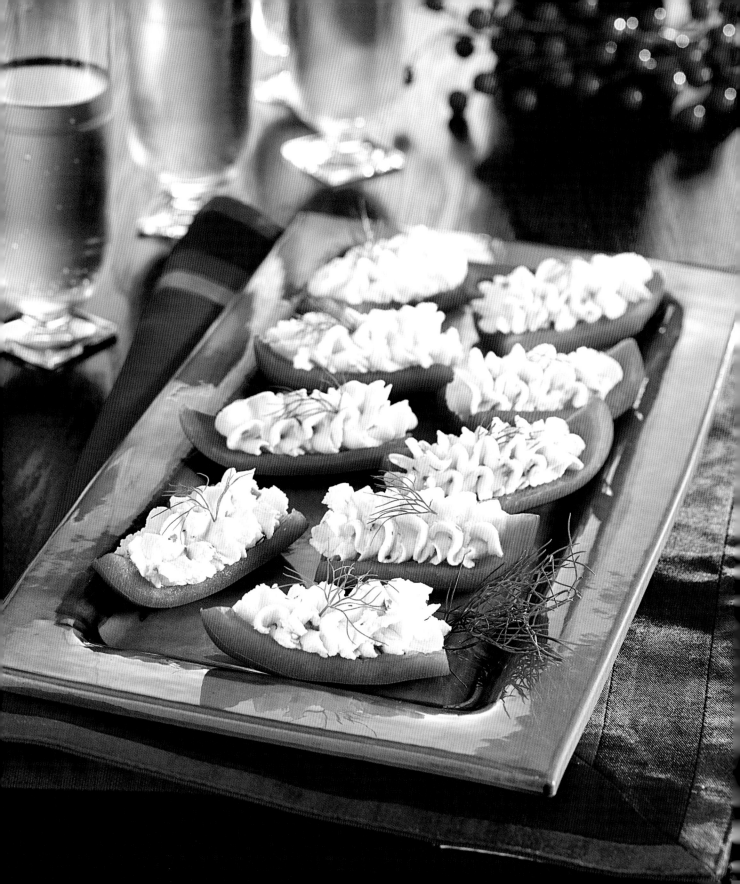

Dill Deviled Eggs

makes 6 servings

PER SERVING

93 calories
6g **total fat**
1g **carbs**
0g **net carbs**
1g **dietary fiber**
7g **protein**

6 **eggs**

1 **tablespoon sour cream**

1 **tablespoon mayonnaise**

1 **tablespoon cottage cheese**

1 **tablespoon minced fresh dill** *or*
   1 teaspoon dried dill weed

1 **tablespoon minced dill pickle**

1 **teaspoon Dijon mustard**

⅛ **teaspoon salt**

⅛ **teaspoon white pepper**
   Paprika (optional)

1. Bring medium saucepan of water to a boil. Gently add eggs with slotted spoon. Reduce heat to maintain a gentle boil; cook 12 minutes. Meanwhile, fill medium bowl with cold water and ice cubes. Drain eggs and place in ice water; cool 10 minutes.

2. Carefully peel eggs. Cut eggs in half; place yolks in small bowl. Add sour cream, mayonnaise, cottage cheese, dill, pickle, mustard, salt and pepper to yolks; mash until well blended.

3. Fill egg halves with yolk mixture. Garnish with paprika.

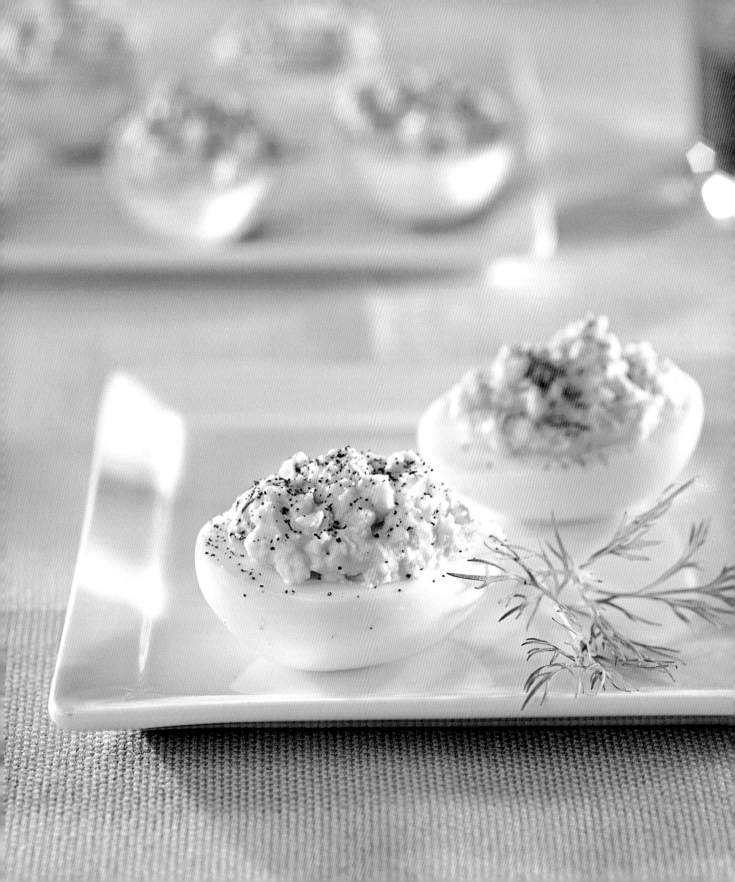

Shrimp, Goat Cheese and Leek Tortilla

makes 6 servings

8 ounces medium raw shrimp, peeled and deveined

4 tablespoons olive oil, divided

2 cloves garlic, minced

2 leeks, chopped

7 eggs

Salt and black pepper

1 package (3 ounces) goat cheese

Olive oil cooking spray

1. Preheat oven to 350°F. Cut each shrimp into 4 pieces.

2. Heat 2 tablespoons oil in medium skillet with ovenproof handle over medium-high heat. Add garlic; cook and stir 30 seconds or just until fragrant. Add shrimp; cook and stir 3 to 4 minutes or until shrimp are pink and opaque. Transfer to plate; set aside.

3. Heat remaining 2 tablespoons oil in same skillet over medium heat. Add leeks; cook and stir 4 to 5 minutes or until tender. Transfer to plate with shrimp; cool 5 minutes.

4. Whisk eggs in medium bowl; season with salt and pepper. Crumble goat cheese into eggs. Stir in shrimp and leeks.

5. Spray same skillet with cooking spray; heat over medium-low heat. Add egg mixture; cook 5 minutes or until edges begin to set. Transfer skillet to oven; bake 10 to 12 minutes or until surface is puffy and center is just set. Remove; cool 10 minutes. Cut into wedges; serve warm or at room temperature.

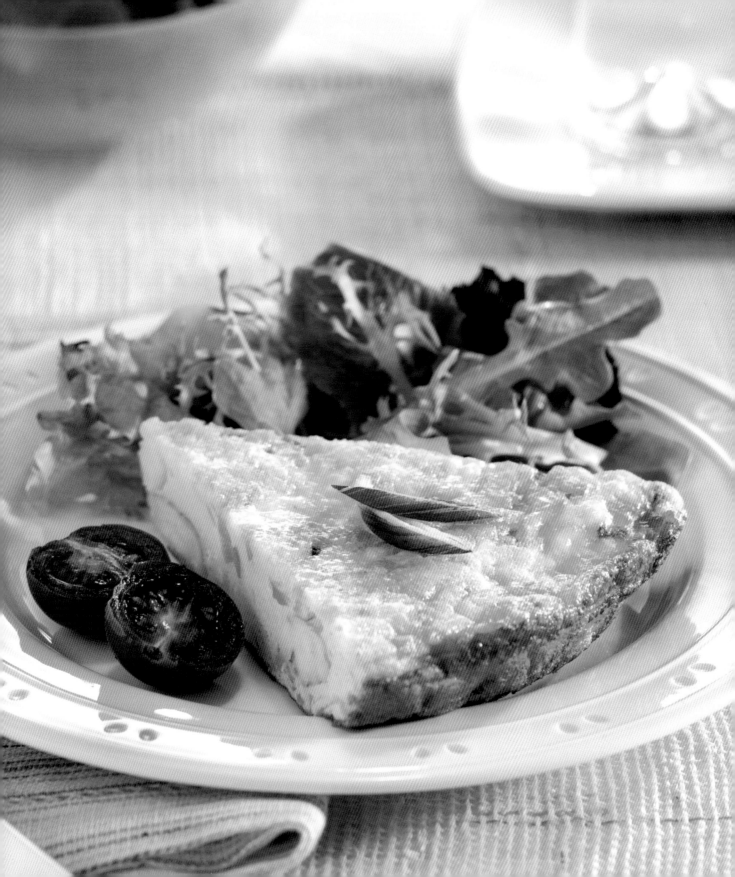

Tuna Salad Stuffed Eggs

makes 4 servings (2 filled eggs per serving)

8 eggs

2 cans (5 ounces each) tuna packed in water, drained

½ cup diced celery

¼ cup mayonnaise

3 tablespoons drained pickle relish

2 tablespoons minced onion

¼ teaspoon lemon-pepper seasoning

⅛ teaspoon salt

1. Bring medium saucepan of water to a boil. Gently add eggs with slotted spoon. Reduce heat to maintain a gentle boil; cook 12 minutes. Meanwhile, fill medium bowl with cold water and ice cubes. Drain eggs and place in ice water; cool 10 minutes.

2. Carefully peel eggs. Cut eggs in half; place 4 yolks in medium bowl (discard remaining yolks). Add tuna, celery, mayonnaise, relish, onion, lemon-pepper and salt; stir until blended.

3. Carefully spoon heaping tablespoon tuna mixture into each egg white. Place filled egg halves together, forming complete egg. Press gently to adhere. Cover and refrigerate at least 2 hours or up to 24 hours.

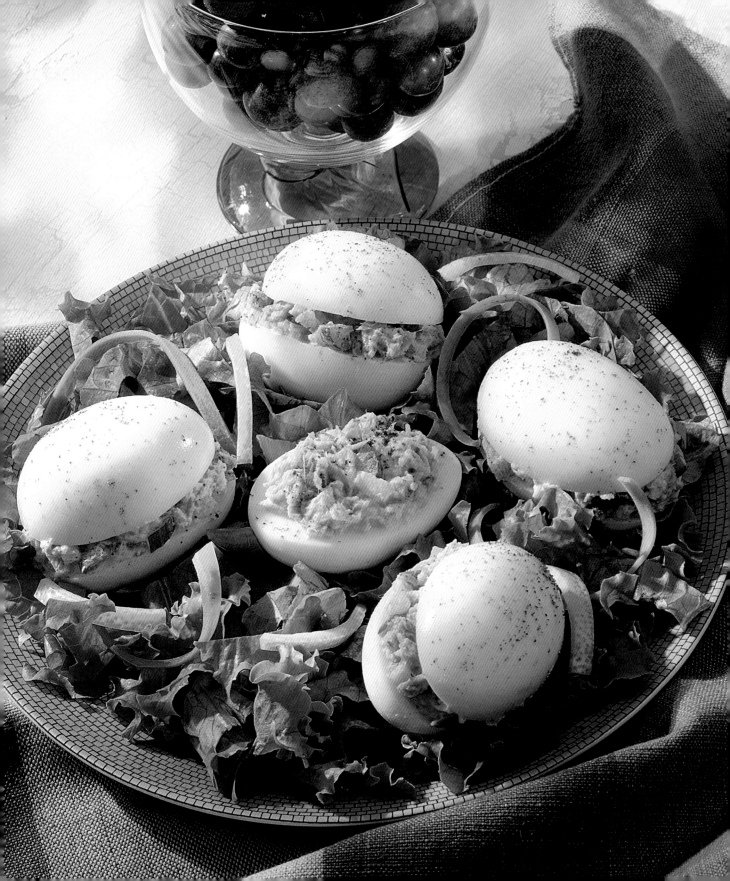

Salmon Celery Trees

makes 12 servings

PER SERVING

60 calories
5g total fat
3g carbs
2g net carbs
1g dietary fiber
3g protein

1 can (6 ounces) pink salmon

2 tablespoons minced fresh dill

1 tablespoon minced green onion

1 tablespoon lemon juice

6 ounces cream cheese, softened

Salt and black pepper

12 celery stalks

Fresh dill sprigs, 3 to 4 inches long (optional)

1. Combine salmon, minced dill, green onion and lemon juice in medium bowl until well blended. Add cream cheese; mash with fork until mixture is smooth. Season to taste with salt and pepper.

2. Stack celery stalks in pairs. Cut each pair into 3-inch pieces.

3. Spread 2 tablespoons salmon mixture into hollowed section of each celery piece. If desired, press dill springs into one half of each celery pair before pressing filled sides together. Stand upright on serving platter with dill sprigs on top to resemble trees.

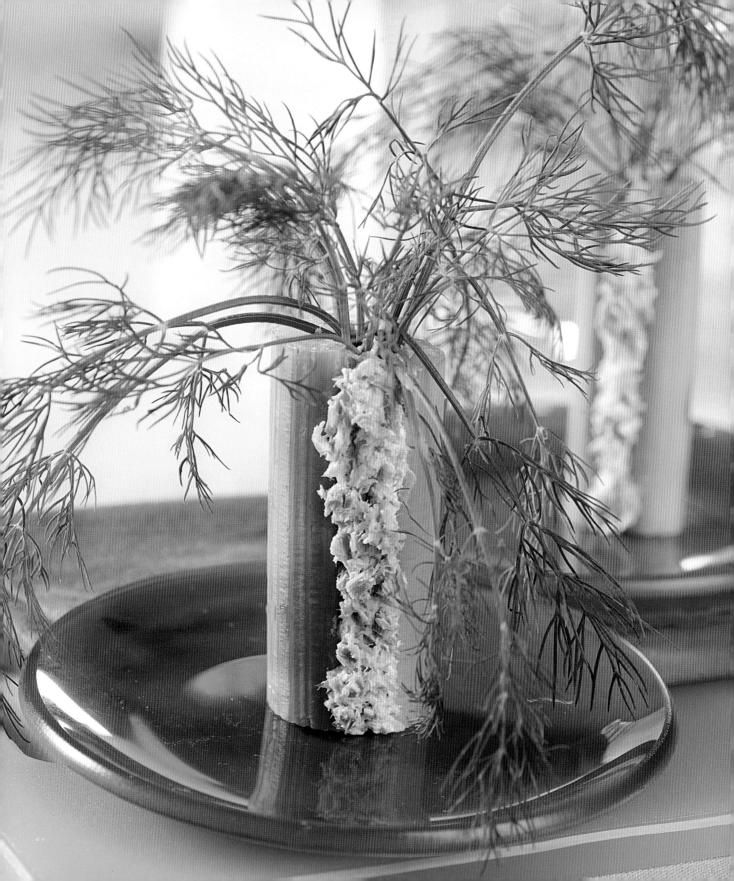

Crab Canapés

makes 16 servings

PER SERVING

58 calories
4g **total fat**
4g **carbs**
3g **net carbs**
1g **dietary fiber**
4g **protein**

⅔ cup cream cheese, softened

2 teaspoons lemon juice

1 teaspoon hot pepper sauce

1 package (8 ounces) imitation crabmeat or lobster, flaked

⅓ cup chopped red bell pepper

2 green onions, sliced (about ¼ cup)

64 cucumber slices (about 2½ medium cucumbers cut into ¼-inch-thick slices)

Chopped fresh parsley (optional)

1. Combine cream cheese, lemon juice and hot pepper sauce in medium bowl; mix well. Stir in crabmeat, bell pepper and green onions. Cover and refrigerate at least 1 hour for flavors to blend.

2. Just before serving, spoon 1½ teaspoons crabmeat mixture onto each cucumber slice. Garnish with parsley.

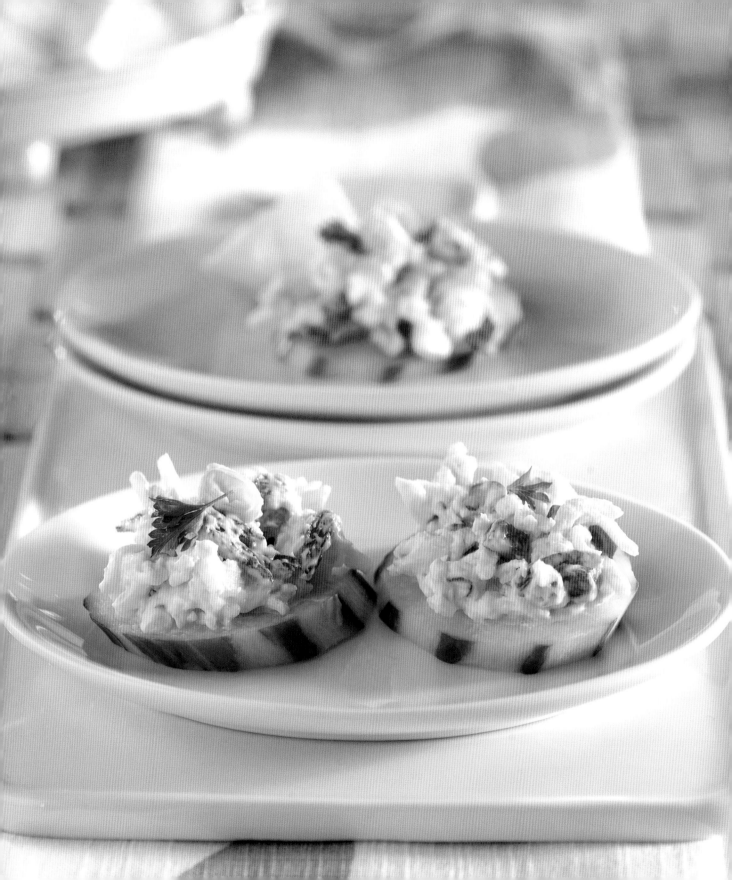

Mozzarella and Prosciutto Bites

makes 16 pieces

PER SERVING

50 calories
4g total fat
0g carbs
0g net carbs
0g dietary fiber
4g protein

16 to 20 small bamboo skewers or toothpicks

8 ounces fresh mozzarella

¼ cup chopped fresh basil

½ teaspoon black pepper

6 thin slices prosciutto

1. Soak skewers in water 20 minutes to prevent burning. Cut mozzarella into 16 (1- to 1½-inch) chunks.* Place on paper towel-lined plate; sprinkle with basil and pepper, turning to coat all sides.

2. Cut prosciutto slices crosswise into thirds. Tightly wrap one slice prosciutto around each piece of mozzarella, covering completely. Insert skewer into each piece. Freeze skewers 15 minutes to firm.

3. Preheat broiler. Line broiler pan or baking sheet with foil. Place skewers on prepared pan; broil about 3 minutes or until prosciutto begins to crisp, turning once. Serve immediately.

*Or substitute one 8-ounce container of small fresh mozzarella balls (ciliengini). One 8-ounce container contains 24 balls.

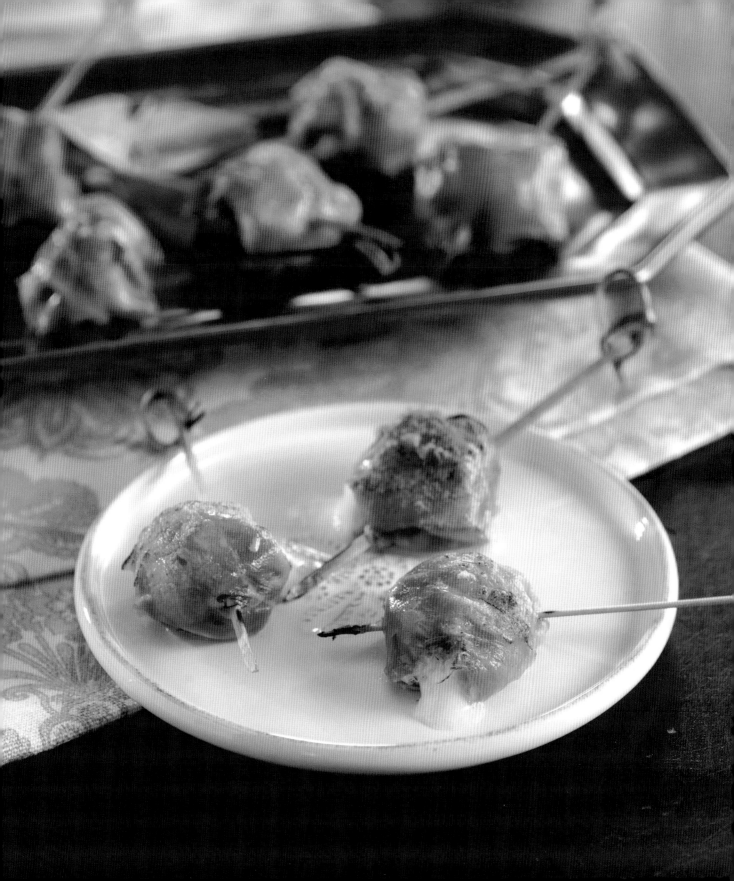

Taco Dip

makes 10 servings

PER SERVING

210 **calories**
19g **total fat**
5g **carbs**
4g **net carbs**
1g **dietary fiber**
9g **protein**

12 ounces cream cheese, softened

½ cup sour cream

2 teaspoons chili powder

1½ teaspoons ground cumin

⅛ teaspoon ground red pepper

½ cup salsa

1 cup (4 ounces) shredded Cheddar cheese

1 cup (4 ounces) shredded Monterey Jack cheese

½ cup diced plum tomatoes

⅓ cup sliced green onions

¼ cup sliced pitted black olives

¼ cup sliced pimiento-stuffed green olives

Shredded lettuce

1. Combine cream cheese, sour cream, chili powder, cumin and red pepper in large bowl; mix until well blended. Stir in salsa.

2. Spread dip on serving platter. Top with cheeses, tomatoes, green onions and olives. Sprinkle shredded lettuce around edges of dip.

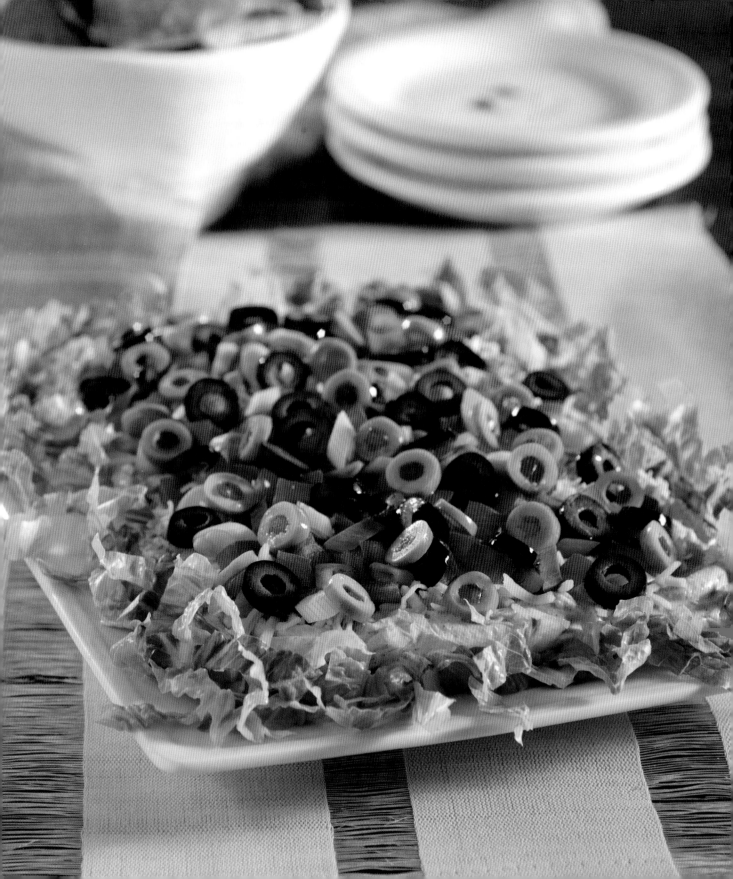

Mediterranean Baked Feta

makes 4 servings

PER SERVING

200 calories
20g total fat
5g carbs
5g net carbs
0g dietary fiber
8g protein

- 1 package (8 ounces) feta cheese, cut crosswise into 4 slices
- ½ cup grape tomatoes, halved
- ¼ cup sliced roasted peppers
- ¼ cup pitted kalamata olives
- ⅛ teaspoon dried oregano
- Black pepper
- 2 tablespoons extra virgin olive oil
- 1 tablespoon shredded fresh basil

1. Preheat oven to 400°F.

2. Place cheese in small baking dish; top with tomatoes, roasted peppers and olives. Sprinkle with oregano and season with black pepper; drizzle with oil.

3. Bake 12 minutes or until cheese is soft. Sprinkle with basil. Serve immediately.

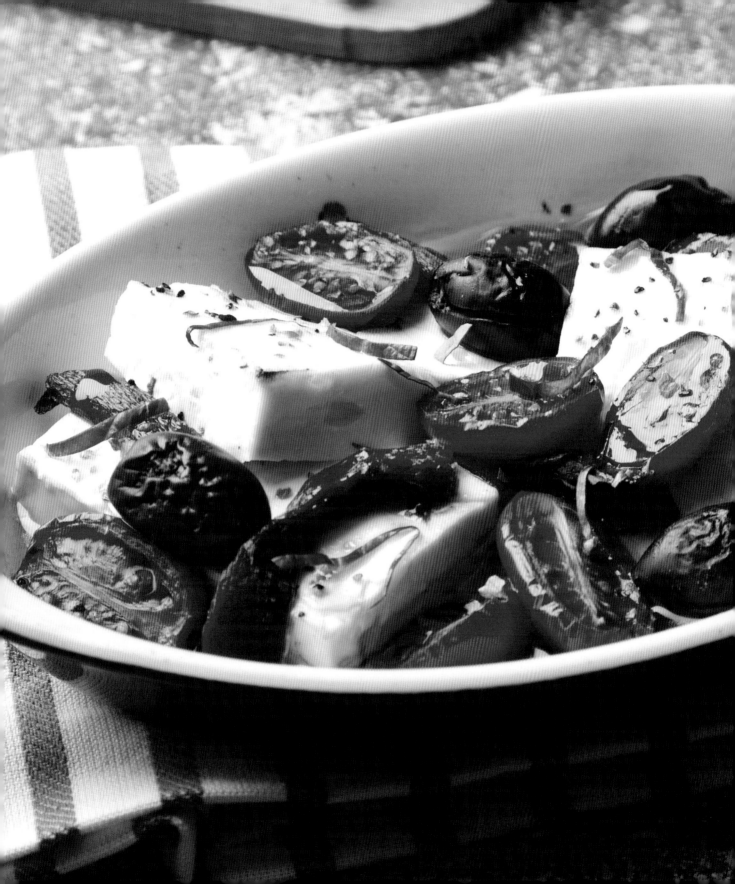

Roasted Red Pepper Dip

makes 2 cups (2 tablespoons per serving)

2 jars (12 ounces each) roasted red peppers in water, drained

1 cup crumbled feta cheese

¼ cup chopped fresh basil

¼ cup sour cream

3 tablespoons Worcestershire sauce

4 cloves garlic

Assorted cut-up fresh vegetables

1. Place roasted red peppers in food processor or blender; process until coarsely chopped. Add cheese, basil, sour cream, Worcestershire sauce and garlic; process until smooth and well blended. Cover and refrigerate at least 2 hours or until chilled.

2. Serve with vegetables.

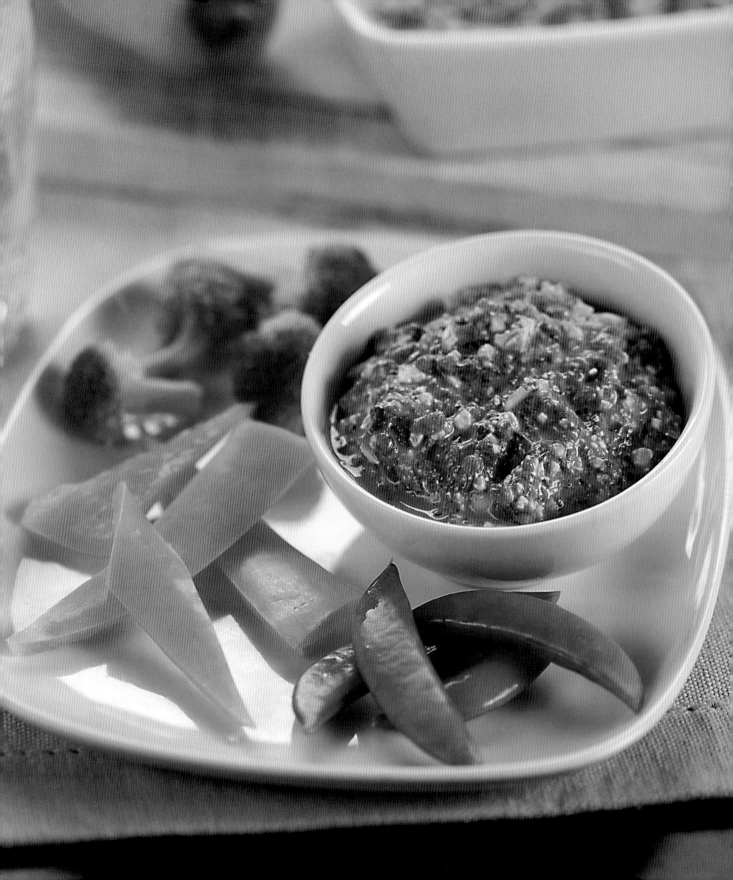

Savory Zucchini Sticks

makes 4 servings

PER SERVING

120 calories
8g **total fat**
6g **carbs**
4g **net carbs**
2g **dietary fiber**
7g **protein**

- 6 tablespoons almond flour
- ¼ cup grated Parmesan cheese
- 1 egg white
- 1 tablespoon water
- 2 small zucchini (about 4 ounces each), cut lengthwise into quarters
- ⅓ cup pasta sauce, warmed

1. Preheat oven to 400°F. Spray baking sheet with nonstick cooking spray.

2. Combine almond flour and cheese in shallow dish. Combine egg white and water in another shallow dish; beat with fork until well blended.

3. Dip each piece of zucchini into egg white mixture, letting excess drip back into dish. Roll in cheese mixture to coat. Place zucchini sticks on prepared baking sheet; spray with cooking spray.

4. Bake 15 to 18 minutes or until golden brown. Serve with pasta sauce.

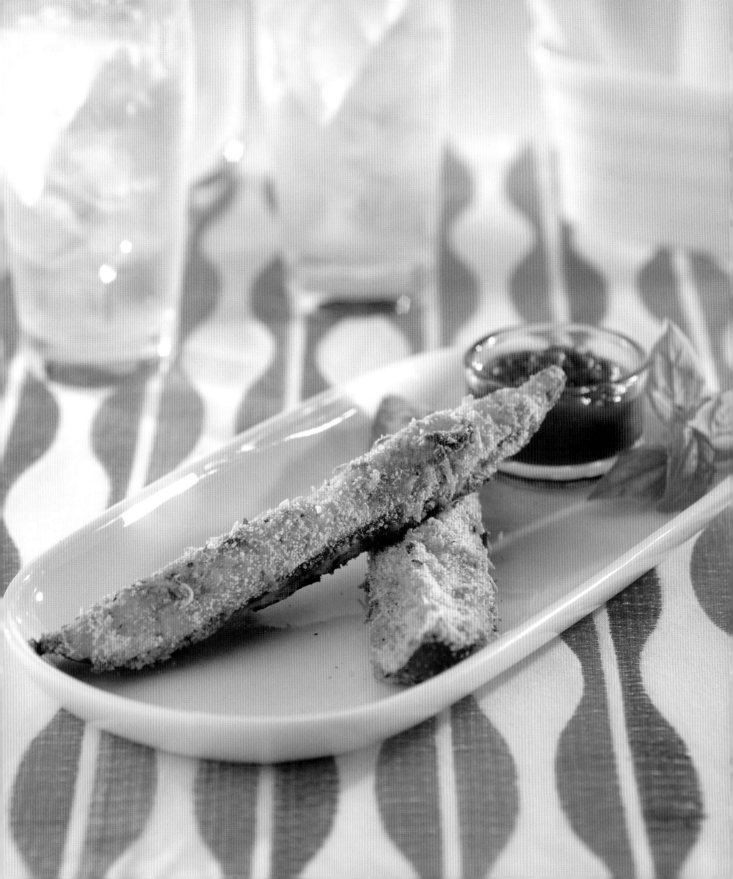

Crab Dip

makes 14 servings (¼ cup per serving)

PER SERVING

110 calories
9g **total fat**
2g **carbs**
2g **net carbs**
0g **dietary fiber**
6g **protein**

½ (8-ounce) package cream cheese, softened

½ cup sour cream

2 tablespoons mayonnaise

¾ teaspoon seasoned salt

¼ teaspoon paprika, plus additional for garnish

2 cans (6 ounces each) crabmeat, drained and flaked

½ cup (2 ounces) shredded mozzarella cheese

2 tablespoons minced onion

2 tablespoons finely chopped green bell pepper*

Chopped fresh parsley (optional)

For a spicier dip, substitute 1 tablespoon minced jalapeño pepper for the bell pepper.

1. Preheat oven to 350°F.

2. Combine cream cheese, sour cream, mayonnaise, seasoned salt and ¼ teaspoon paprika in medium bowl; stir until well blended and smooth. Add crabmeat, mozzarella cheese, onion and bell pepper; stir until blended. Spread in small (1-quart) shallow baking dish.

3. Bake 15 to 20 minutes or until bubbly and top is beginning to brown. Garnish with additional paprika and parsley.

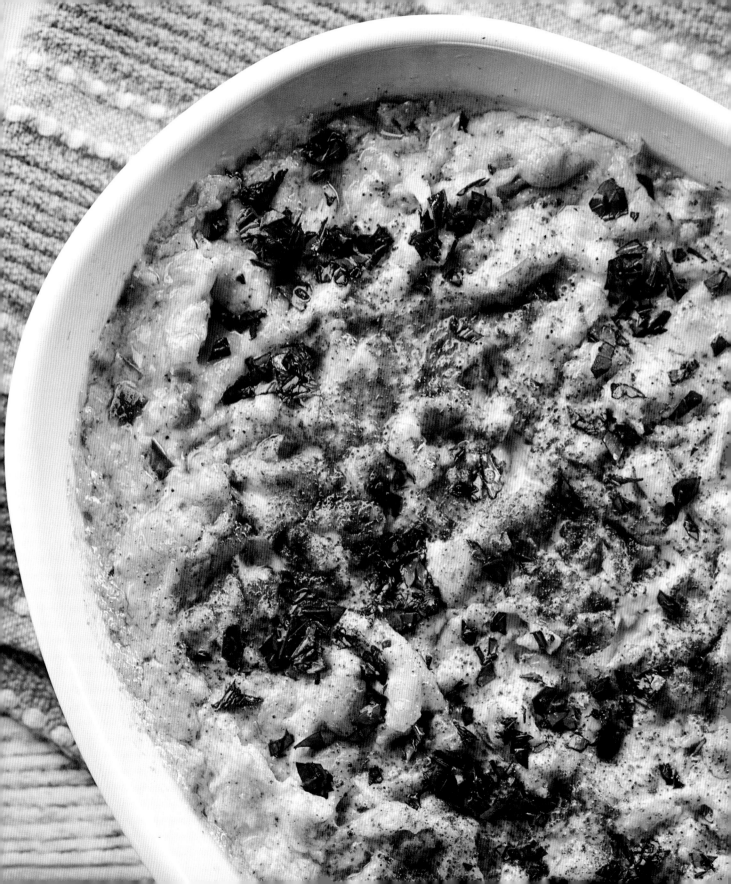

Classic Deviled Eggs

makes 12 deviled eggs (1 per serving)

PER SERVING

30 calories
3g **total fat**
0g **carbs**
0g **net carbs**
0g **dietary fiber**
2g **protein**

6 eggs

3 tablespoons mayonnaise

½ teaspoon apple cider vinegar

½ teaspoon yellow mustard

⅛ teaspoon salt

   Optional toppings: black pepper, regular or smoked paprika, ground red pepper, drained capers, minced chives and/or minced red onion

1. Bring medium saucepan of water to a boil. Gently add eggs with slotted spoon. Reduce heat to maintain a gentle boil; cook 12 minutes. Meanwhile, fill medium bowl with cold water and ice cubes. Drain eggs and place in ice water; cool 10 minutes.

2. Carefully peel eggs. Cut eggs in half; place yolks in small bowl. Add mayonnaise, vinegar, mustard and salt; mash until well blended. Spoon mixture into egg whites; garnish with desired toppings.

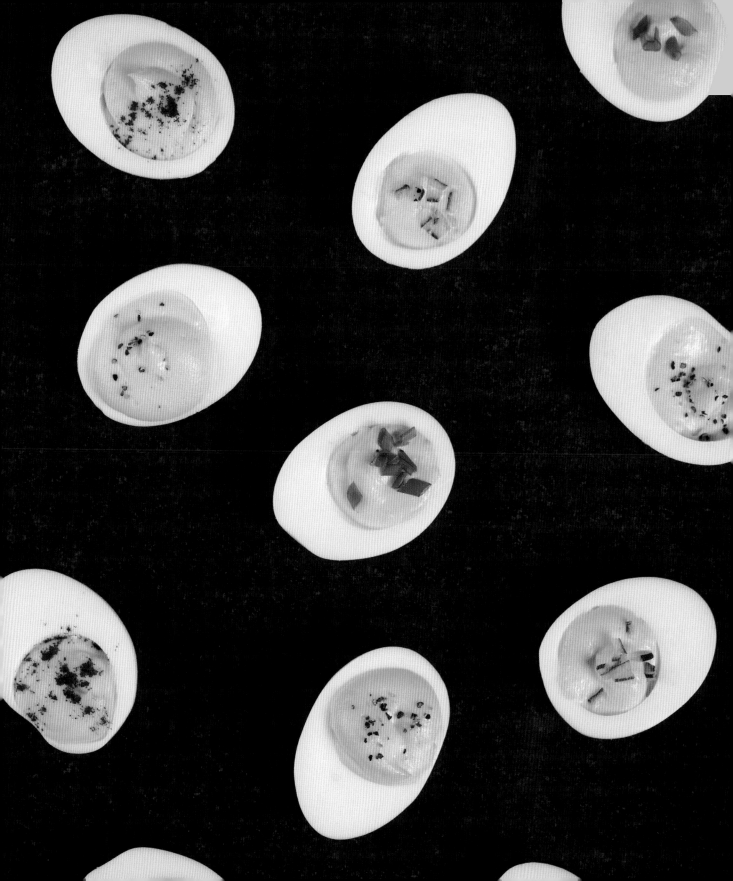

Cherry Tomato Pops

makes 8 pops

4 **mozzarella string cheese sticks
    (1 ounce each)**

8 **cherry tomatoes**

3 **tablespoons ranch dressing**

1. Slice cheese sticks in half lengthwise. Trim stem end of each cherry tomato and remove pulp and seeds.

2. Press end of cheese stick into hollowed tomato to make cherry tomato pop. Serve with ranch dressing for dipping.

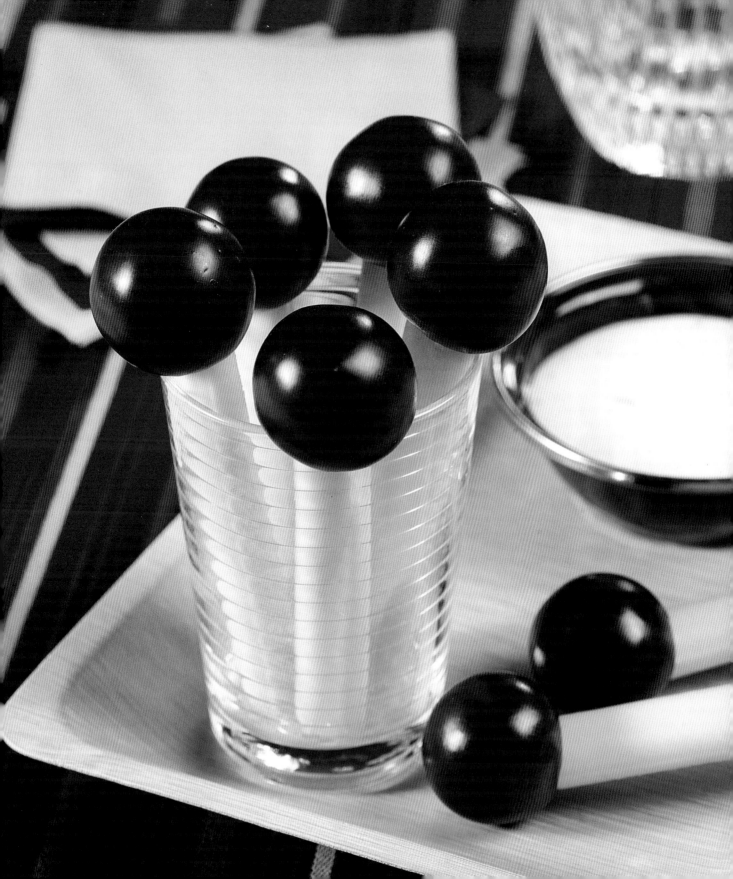

Colorful Kabobs

makes 10 kabobs

PER SERVING

170 **calories**
14g **total fat**
4g **carbs**
3g **net carbs**
1g **dietary fiber**
6g **protein**

30 cocktail-size smoked sausages

20 cherry or grape tomatoes

20 large pimiento-stuffed green olives

2 yellow bell peppers, cut into 1-inch squares

¼ cup (½ stick) butter, melted

Lemon juice (optional)

1. Preheat oven to 450°F.

2. Thread 3 sausages onto 8-inch wooden skewer, alternating with tomatoes, olives and bell peppers. Repeat with remaining ingredients.

3. Place skewers on rack in shallow baking pan. Brush with melted butter and drizzle with lemon juice, if desired. Bake 4 to 6 minutes or until hot.

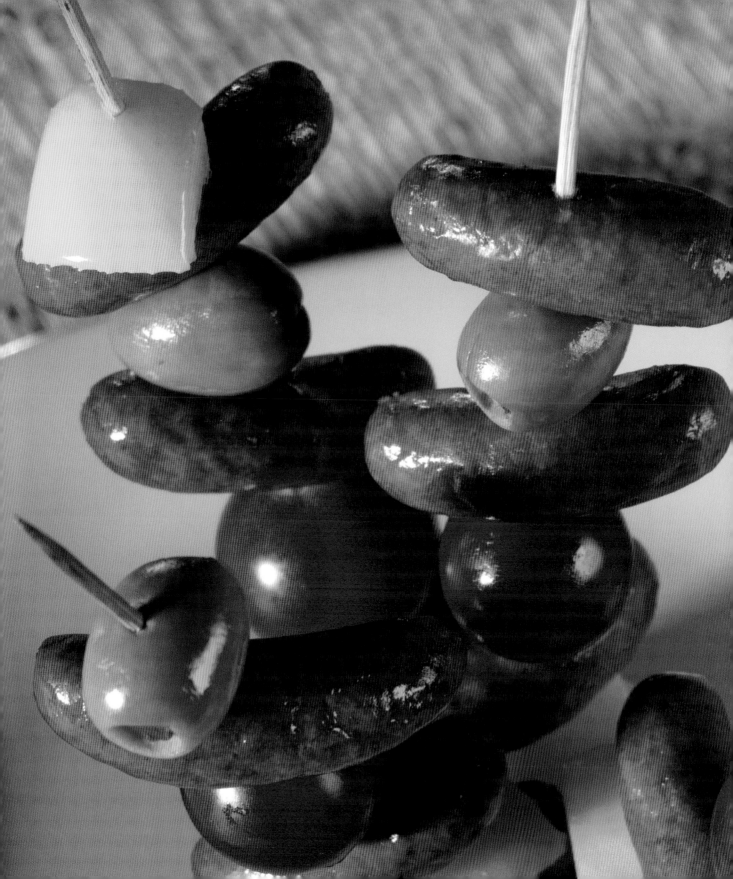

Rosemary Nut Mix

makes 6 cups (3 tablespoons per serving)

2 tablespoons butter

2 cups pecan halves

1 cup unsalted macadamia nuts

1 cup walnuts

1 teaspoon dried rosemary

½ teaspoon salt

¼ teaspoon red pepper flakes

1. Preheat oven to 300°F.

2. Melt butter in large saucepan over low heat. Stir in pecans, macadamia nuts and walnuts. Add rosemary, salt and red pepper flakes; cook and stir about 1 minute. Spread mixture onto ungreased baking sheet.

3. Bake 15 minutes, stirring occasionally. Cool completely on baking sheet on wire rack.

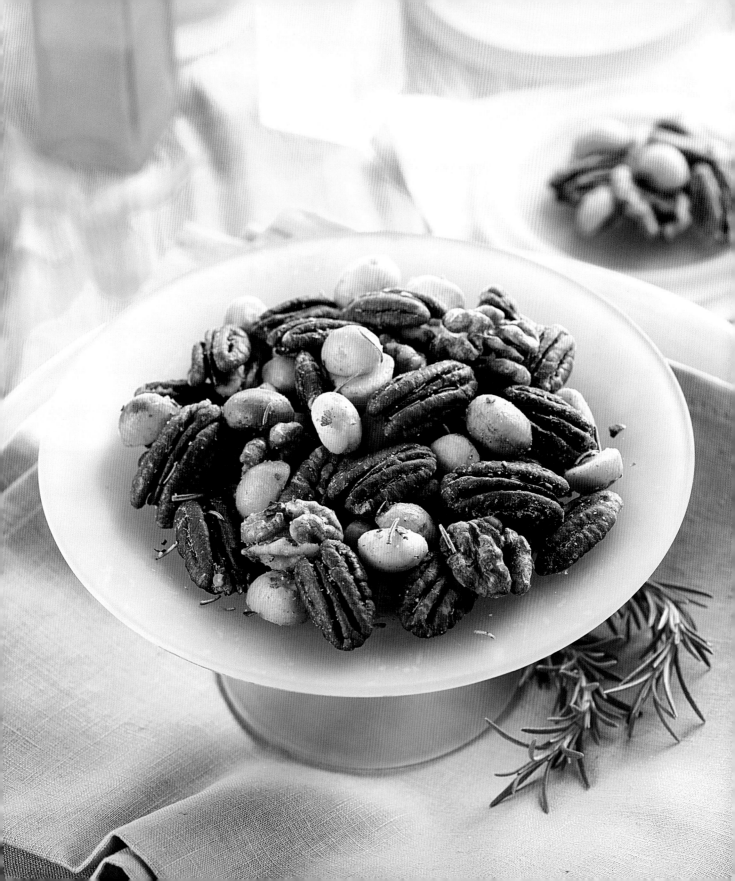

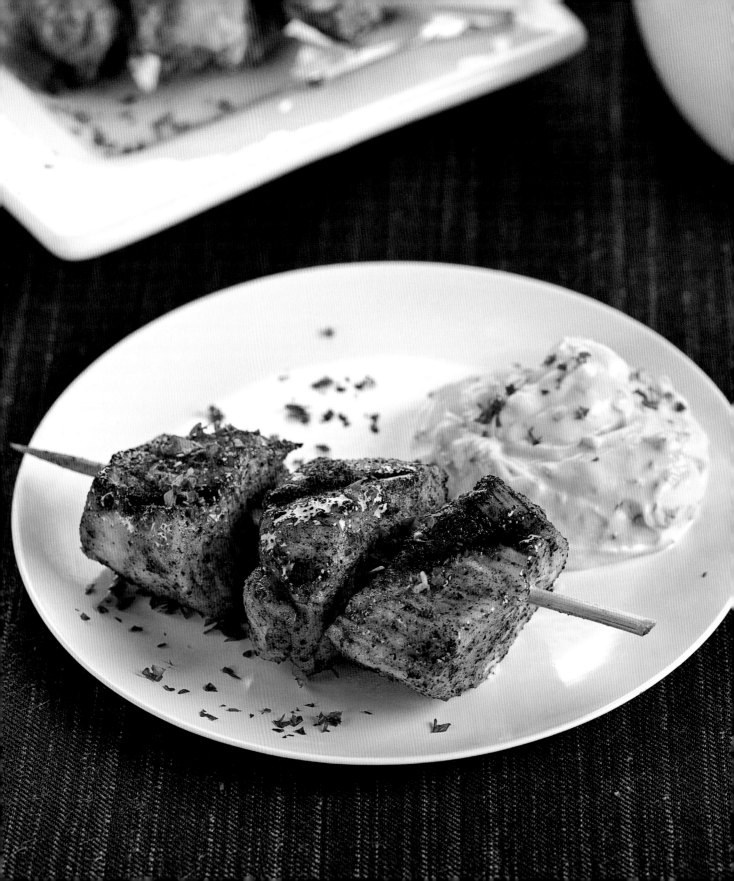

chicken *and* turkey

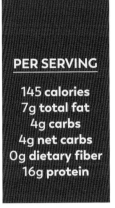
Spiced Chicken Skewers with Yogurt-Tahini Sauce

makes 8 servings

- 1 cup plain nonfat or regular Greek yogurt
- ¼ cup chopped fresh parsley, plus additional for garnish
- ¼ cup tahini
- 2 tablespoons lemon juice
- 1 clove garlic
- ¾ teaspoon salt, divided
- 1 tablespoon vegetable oil
- 2 teaspoons garam masala
- 1 pound boneless skinless chicken breasts, cut into 1-inch pieces

1. Spray grid with nonstick cooking spray. Prepare grill for direct cooking.

2. For sauce, combine yogurt, ¼ cup parsley, tahini, lemon juice, garlic and ¼ teaspoon salt in food processor or blender; process until smooth. Set aside.

3. Combine oil, garam masala and remaining ½ teaspoon salt in medium bowl. Add chicken; toss to coat. Thread chicken on eight 6-inch wooden or metal skewers.

4. Grill chicken skewers over medium-high heat 5 minutes per side or until chicken is no longer pink. Serve with sauce. Garnish with additional parsley.

Grilled Chicken with Chimichurri Salsa

makes 4 servings

4 boneless skinless chicken breasts (6 ounces each)

½ cup plus 4 teaspoons olive oil, divided

Salt and black pepper

½ cup finely chopped fresh parsley

¼ cup white wine vinegar

2 tablespoons finely chopped onion

3 cloves garlic, minced

1 jalapeño pepper, finely chopped

2 teaspoons dried oregano

1. Prepare grill for direct cooking.

2. Brush chicken with 4 teaspoons oil; season with salt and black pepper. Place on grid over medium heat. Grill, covered, 10 to 16 minutes or until chicken is no longer pink in center (165°F), turning once.

3. For salsa, combine parsley, remaining ½ cup oil, vinegar, onion, garlic, jalapeño and oregano in small bowl. Season with salt and black pepper. Serve over chicken.

Tip: Chimichurri salsa has a fresh, green color. Serve it with grilled steak or fish as well as chicken. Chimichurri will remain fresh tasting for 24 hours.

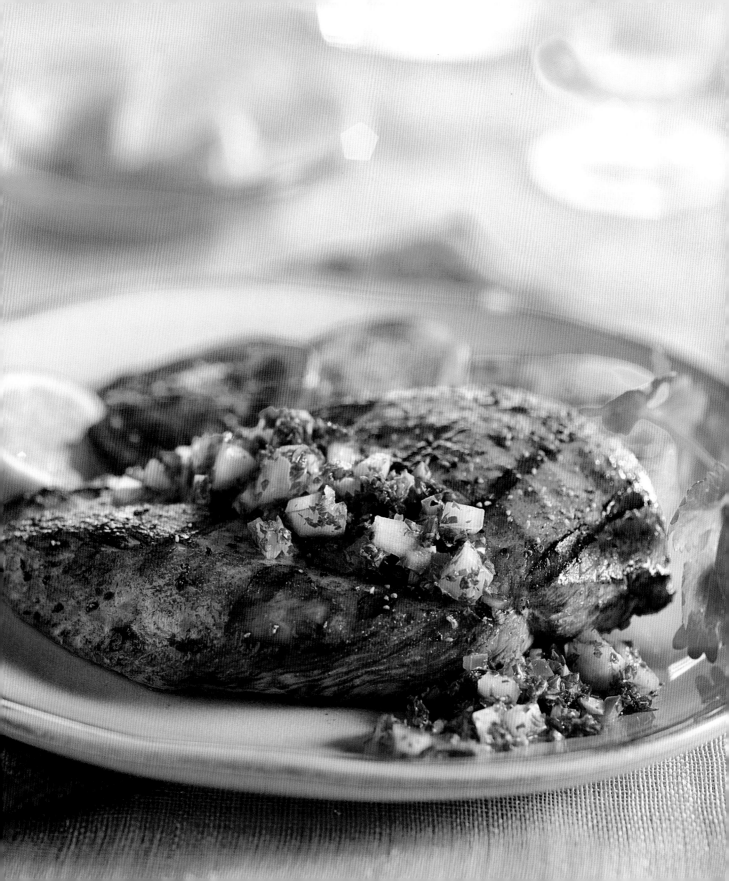

Cajun Chicken Drums

makes 2 servings

PER SERVING

173 calories
5g **total fat**
2g **carbs**
1g **net carbs**
1g **dietary fiber**
29g **protein**

4 chicken drumsticks, skin removed

½ teaspoon Cajun seasoning

2 tablespoons lemon juice

½ teaspoon grated lemon peel

½ teaspoon salt

½ teaspoon hot pepper sauce

2 tablespoons chopped fresh parsley (optional)

1. Preheat oven to 400°F. Spray shallow baking dish with nonstick cooking spray. Arrange chicken in dish; sprinkle evenly with Cajun seasoning. Cover dish with foil; bake 25 minutes, turning drumsticks once.

2. Remove foil; bake 15 to 20 minutes or until cooked through and juices run clear (165°F). Remove from oven. Stir in lemon juice, lemon peel, salt and hot pepper sauce; toss to blend, scraping bottom and sides of baking dish. Sprinkle with parsley, if desired. Serve immediately.

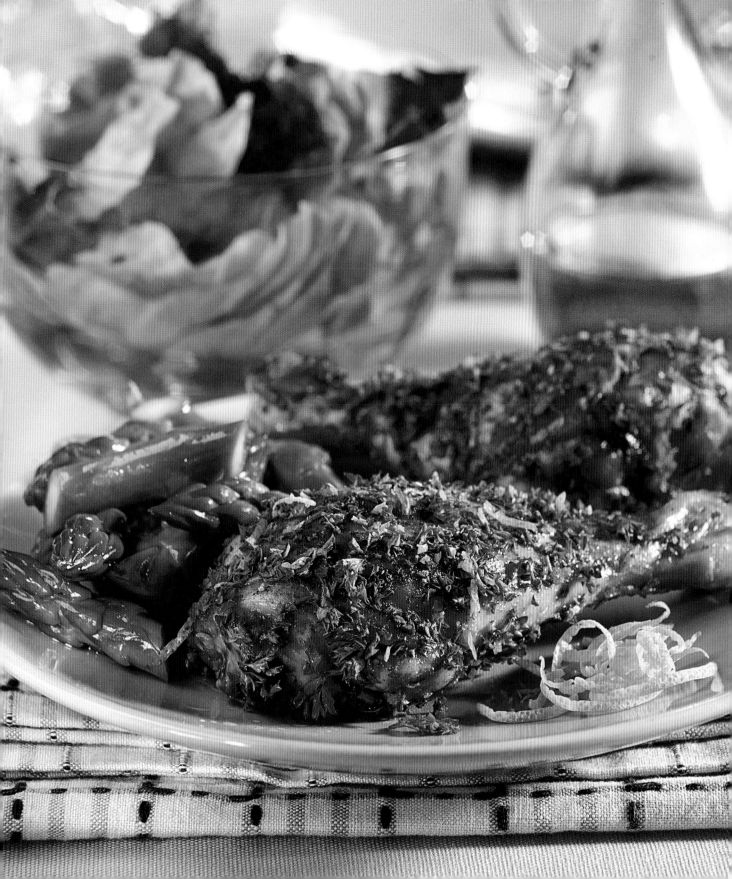

Braised Chicken with Vegetables

makes 4 servings

PER SERVING

177 calories
5g **total fat**
6g **carbs**
4g **net carbs**
2g **dietary fiber**
24g **protein**

4 chicken drumsticks, skin removed

1 cup chicken broth

2 tablespoons lemon juice

1½ tablespoons salt-free seasoning blend

2 cloves garlic, minced

½ teaspoon dried rosemary

¼ teaspoon smoked paprika

2 cups assorted chopped vegetables (such as yellow squash, zucchini, onion and/or bell peppers)

Salt

1. Combine chicken, broth and lemon juice in large skillet. Cover and cook over medium heat 15 minutes, turning chicken occasionally.

2. Add seasoning, garlic, rosemary and paprika; cook and stir 1 minute. Add vegetables; cover and cook 10 to 15 minutes or until chicken is cooked through (165°F) and vegetables are tender. Season with salt, if desired.

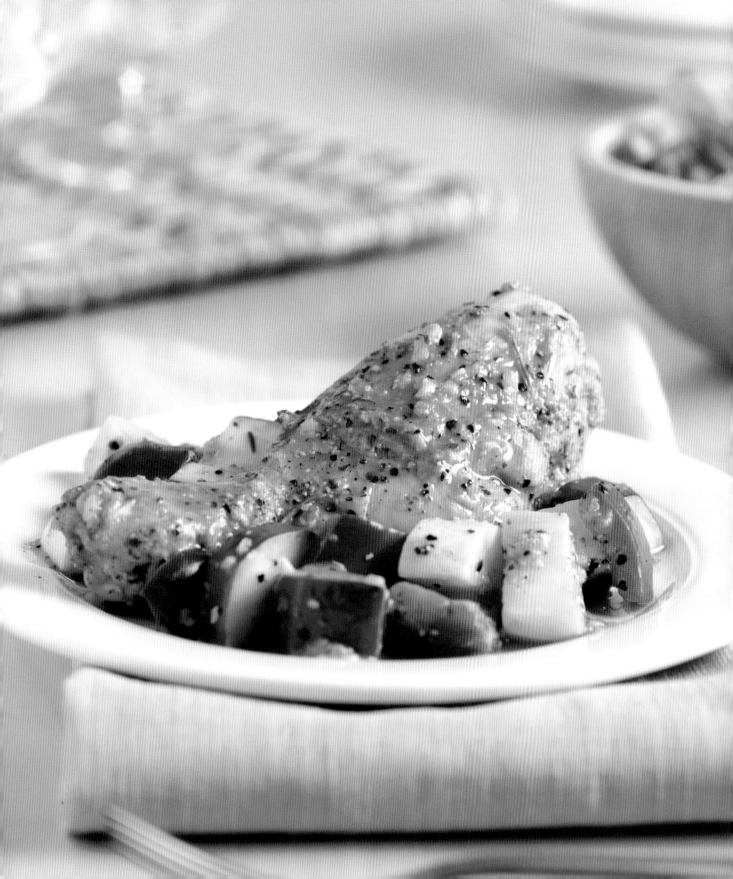

Pesto-Stuffed Grilled Chicken

makes 6 servings

PER SERVING

280 calories
18g **total fat**
4g **carbs**
4g **net carbs**
0g **dietary fiber**
25g **protein**

2 cloves garlic, peeled

½ cup packed fresh basil leaves

2 tablespoons pine nuts or walnuts, toasted*

¼ teaspoon black pepper

5 tablespoons extra virgin olive oil, divided

¼ cup grated Parmesan cheese

1 fresh or thawed frozen roasting chicken or capon (6 to 7 pounds)

2 tablespoons fresh lemon juice

To toast pine nuts, spread in single layer in small heavy skillet. Cook and stir 2 to 3 minutes or until golden brown, stirring frequently.

1. Prepare grill with metal or foil drip pan. Bank briquettes on either side of drip pan for indirect cooking.

2. For pesto, drop garlic through feed tube of food processor with motor running. Add basil, pine nuts and black pepper; process until basil is minced. With motor running, add 3 tablespoons oil in thin steady stream until smooth paste forms, scraping down side of bowl once. Add cheese; process until well blended.

3. Remove giblets from chicken cavity; reserve for another use. Loosen skin over breast of chicken by pushing fingers between skin and meat, taking care not to tear skin. Do not loosen skin over wings and drumsticks. Using rubber spatula or small spoon, spread pesto under breast skin; massage skin to evenly spread pesto. Combine remaining 2 tablespoons oil and lemon juice in small bowl; brush over chicken skin. Tuck wings under back; tie legs together with kitchen string.

4. Place chicken, breast side up, on grid directly over drip pan. Grill, covered, over medium-low coals 1 hour 10 minutes to 1 hour 30 minutes or until thermometer inserted into thickest part of thigh not touching bone registers 185°F, adding 4 to 9 briquettes to both sides of the fire after 45 minutes to maintain medium-low coals. Transfer chicken to large cutting board; tent with foil. Let stand 15 minutes before carving.

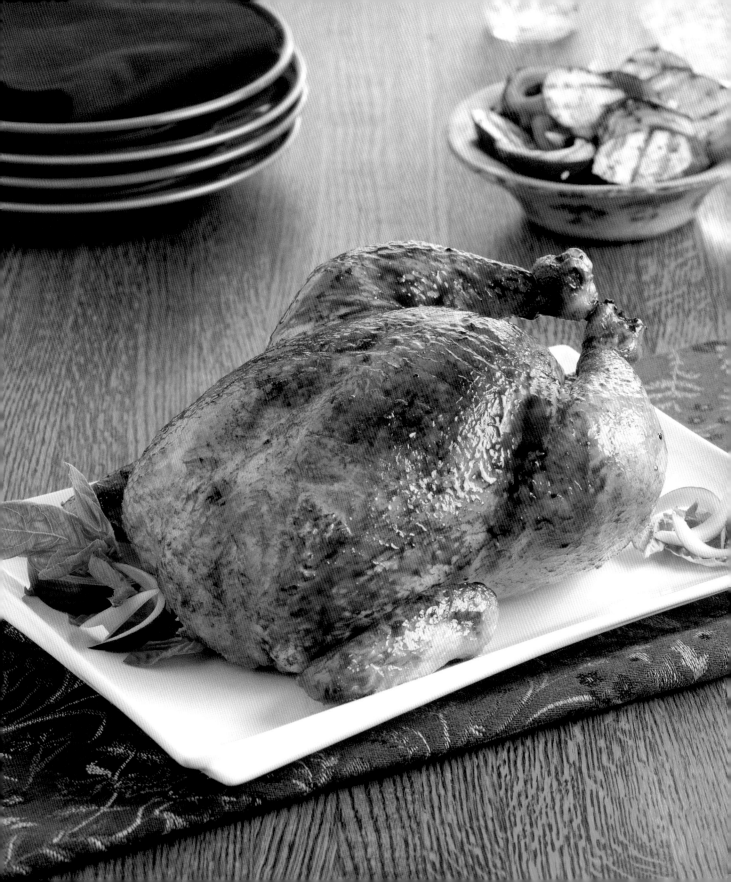

Asparagus and Cheddar Stuffed Chicken Breasts

makes 4 servings

20 asparagus spears (about 2 bunches)

2 cups chicken broth

1 medium red bell pepper, chopped

   Salt and black pepper

½ teaspoon minced garlic

1 teaspoon dried parsley flakes

4 boneless skinless chicken breasts (about 4 ounces each)

4 tablespoons (1 ounce) shredded Cheddar cheese

1. Snap woody stem ends off asparagus and discard. Cut off asparagus tips about 4 inches long; set aside. Slice asparagus stalks and combine with broth, bell pepper, ¼ teaspoon salt, garlic, parsley and ¼ teaspoon black pepper in saucepan. Cook over medium-high heat 10 minutes or until vegetables are tender, stirring occasionally.

2. Meanwhile, place each chicken breast half between plastic wrap and pound with rolling pin until approximately ¼ inch thick. Season chicken with salt and pepper.

3. Preheat electric indoor grill with lid. Lay 5 asparagus tips across one end of each pounded breast. Top each with 1 tablespoon cheese and fold in half. Place stuffed breasts on grill and cook with lid closed for 6 minutes.

4. Spoon vegetable sauce onto serving plates; top with chicken.

Note: If you don't have an electric indoor grill, cook in grill pan or bake in oven on baking sheet at 350°F for 10 minutes or until cooked through.

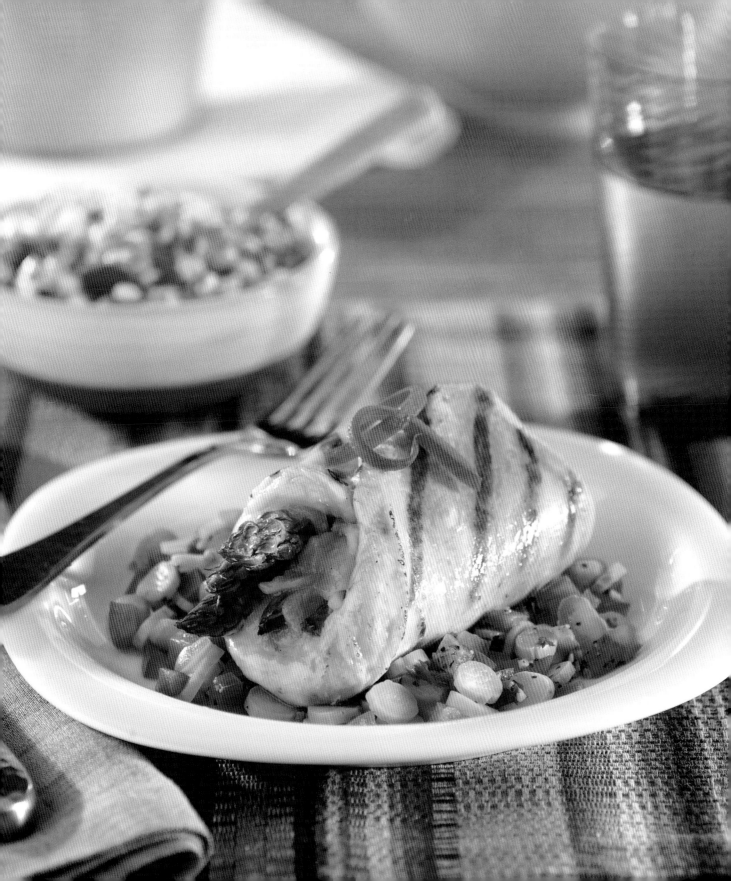

Chicken Cacciatore

makes 6 servings

4 **pounds chicken pieces**

½ **teaspoon salt, divided**

¼ **teaspoon black pepper, divided**

1 **tablespoon olive oil**

1 **medium onion, chopped**

2 **medium red or green bell peppers, cut into strips**

2 **cups sliced mushrooms**

1 **clove garlic, minced**

1 **can (28 ounces) whole tomatoes, undrained**

½ **cup dry red wine**

2 **teaspoons dried basil**

1 **teaspoon dried oregano**

1 **cup (4 ounces) shredded mozzarella cheese**

¼ **cup grated Parmesan cheese**

1. Sprinkle chicken with ¼ teaspoon salt and ⅛ teaspoon black pepper. Heat oil in deep 12-inch skillet over medium heat. Brown chicken on both sides; transfer to plate.

2. Add onion to same skillet; cook and stir over medium heat 3 minutes. Add bell peppers, mushrooms and garlic; cook and stir 3 to 4 minutes or until vegetables are softened. Cut tomatoes into quarters. Add tomatoes with juice, wine, basil, oregano, remaining ¼ teaspoon salt and black pepper. Bring to a boil.

3. Add chicken; reduce heat to low. Cover and cook 25 to 30 minutes or until chicken juices run clear. Remove chicken from skillet; keep warm.

4. Cook tomato mixture, uncovered, over medium heat 5 to 10 minutes or until tomato mixture thickens slightly. Return chicken to skillet; sprinkle with cheeses. Cook briefly until mozzarella cheese melts.

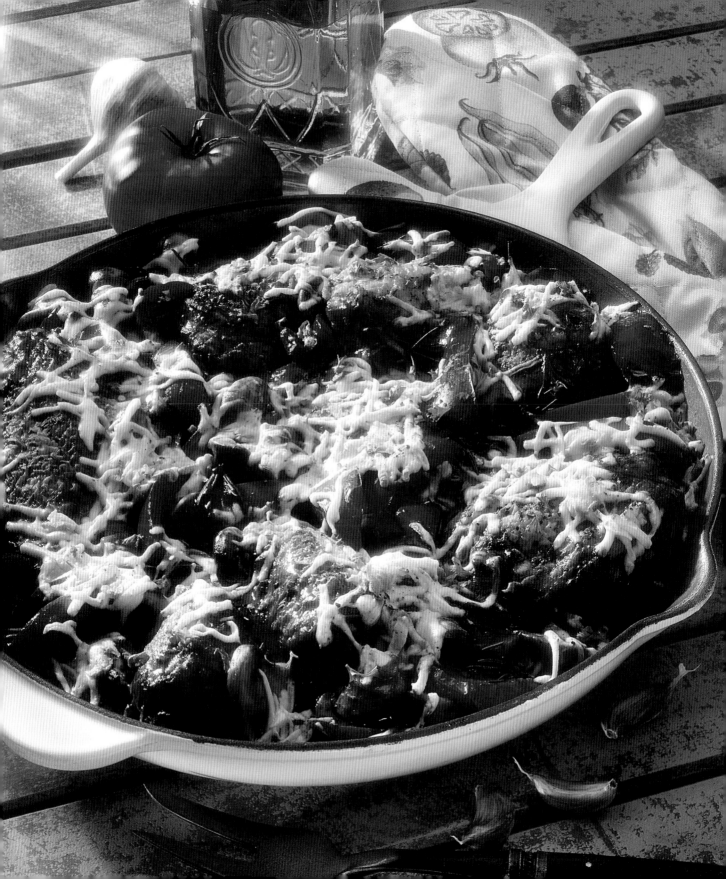

Southwest Chicken Burgers with Avocado Salad

makes 4 servings

- 1 cup finely diced yellow or red bell pepper, divided
- ½ cup finely diced red onion, divided
- 1 egg white
- 1½ teaspoons chili powder, divided
- 20 ounces ground chicken
- 1 medium avocado, diced
- ½ cup finely diced cucumber
- Juice of 1 lime
- 4 tablespoons (1 ounce) shredded Cheddar cheese

1. Combine ½ cup bell pepper, ¼ cup onion, egg white and 1 teaspoon chili powder in large bowl. Add chicken; stir to combine. Shape mixture into 4 patties. Cover and refrigerate 15 minutes.

2. Combine avocado, cucumber, lime juice, remaining ½ cup bell pepper, ¼ cup onion and ½ teaspoon chili powder in medium bowl.

3. Spray large skillet with nonstick cooking spray; heat over medium heat. Add burgers; cook 5 minutes. Turn and top each burger with 1 tablespoon cheese. Cook 5 minutes or until no longer pink in center.

4. Divide avocado salad among serving plates; top with burgers.

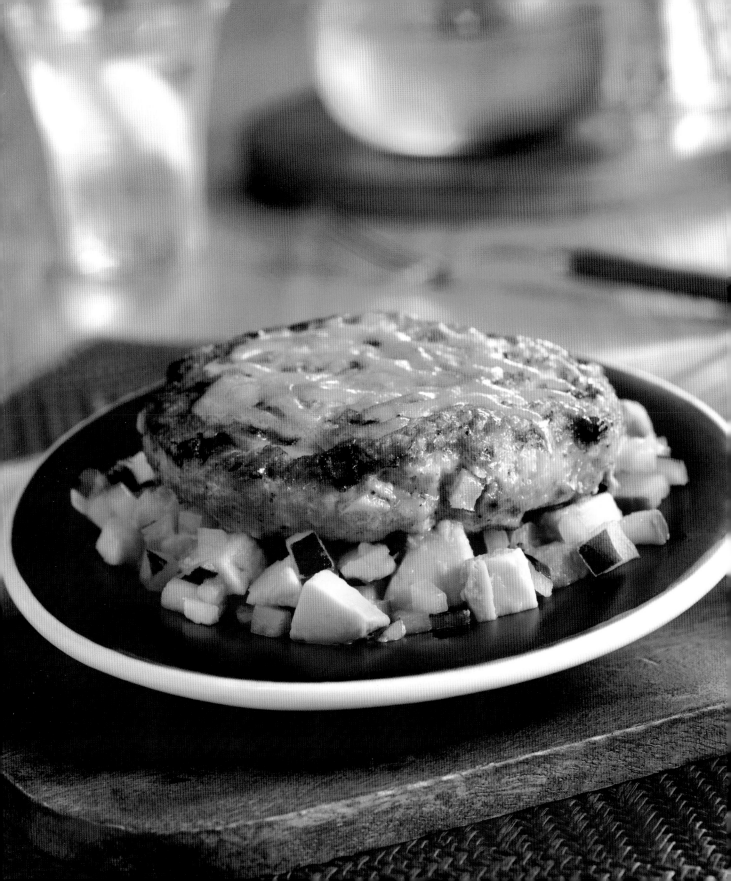

Teriyaki Chicken Drummies

makes 12 servings

PER SERVING

160 **calories**
10g **total fat**
2g **carbs**
2g **net carbs**
0g **dietary fiber**
12g **protein**

1 bottle (10 ounces) teriyaki sauce, divided

4 cloves garlic, crushed

¼ teaspoon black pepper

3 pounds chicken drummettes (about 24 pieces total)

1 tablespoon toasted sesame seeds*

To toast sesame seeds, spread seeds in small skillet. Shake skillet over medium-low heat about 3 minutes or until seeds begin to pop and turn golden.

1. Reserve ¼ cup teriyaki sauce; set aside. Combine remaining teriyaki sauce, garlic and pepper in shallow baking dish. Add drummettes; marinate in refrigerator 30 minutes, turning once.

2. Preheat oven to 400°F. Spray baking sheet with nonstick cooking spray. Place drummettes, skin side up, on prepared baking sheet; discard marinade.

3. Bake 30 minutes or until golden brown. Immediately remove drummettes to large bowl. Add reserved ¼ cup teriyaki sauce; toss to coat evenly. Sprinkle with sesame seeds.

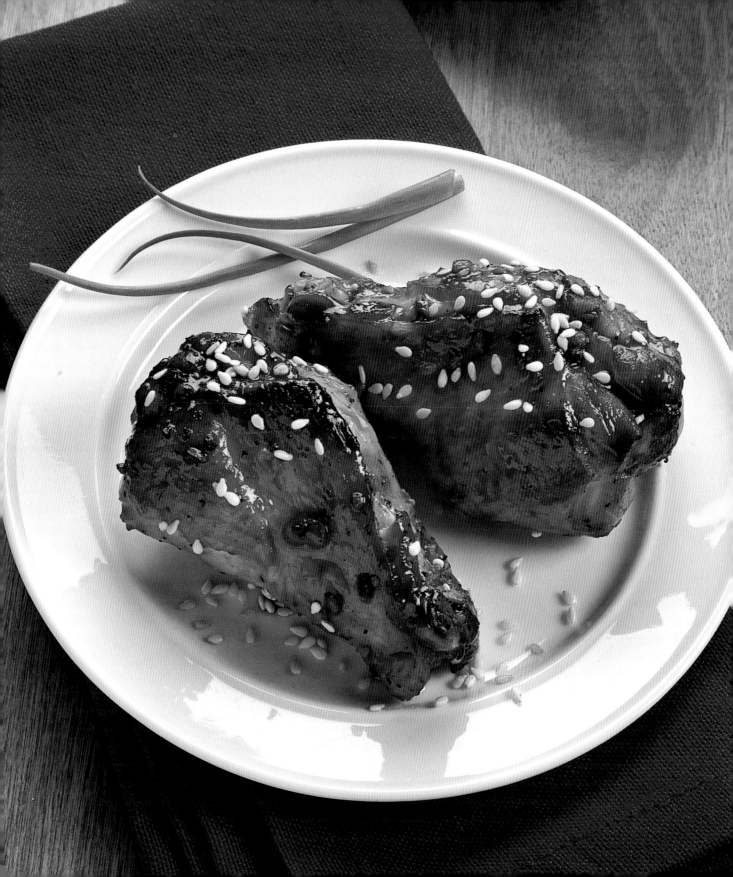

Roast Turkey Breast with Spinach and Blue Cheese Stuffing

makes 14 servings

1 frozen whole boneless turkey breast (3½ to 4 pounds), thawed

1 package (10 ounces) frozen chopped spinach, thawed and squeezed dry

½ cup (2ounces) blue cheese or feta cheese

2 ounces regular cream cheese or Neufchâtel, softened

½ cup finely chopped green onions

1½ tablespoons Dijon mustard

1½ tablespoons dried basil

2 teaspoons dried oregano

Salt, black pepper and paprika

1. Preheat oven to 350°F. Spray roasting pan and rack with nonstick cooking spray.

2. Unroll turkey breast; rinse and pat dry. Place turkey between 2 sheets of plastic wrap or waxed paper. Pound turkey to 1-inch thickness using flat side of meat mallet or rolling pin. Remove and discard skin from one half of turkey breast; turn meat over so skin side faces down.

3. Combine spinach, blue cheese, cream cheese, green onions, mustard, basil and oregano in medium bowl; mix well. Spread evenly over turkey breast. Roll up turkey so skin is on top. Tie closed with kitchen string.

4. Carefully place turkey breast on rack; season with salt, pepper and paprika. Roast 1½ hours or until no longer pink in center of breast (165°F). Remove from oven; let stand 10 minutes. Remove skin and slice into 14 (¼-inch-thick) slices.

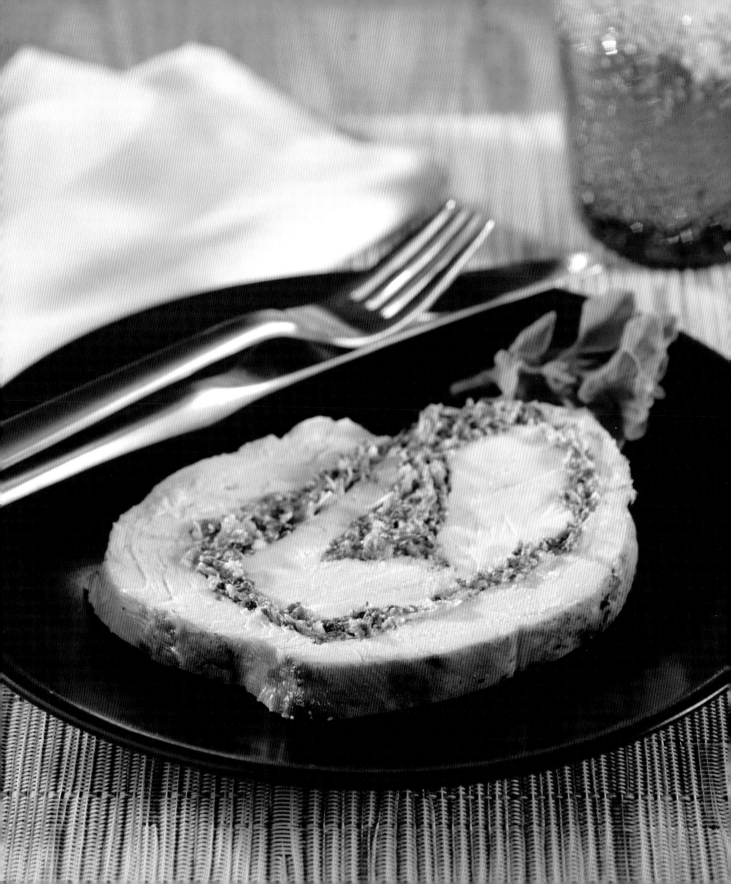

Kung Pao Chicken

makes 3 servings

5 teaspoons dry sherry, divided

5 teaspoons soy sauce, divided

3½ teaspoons coconut flour, divided

¼ teaspoon salt

1 pound boneless skinless chicken breasts, cut into bite-size pieces

2 tablespoons chicken broth or water

1 tablespoon red wine vinegar

3 tablespoons vegetable oil, divided

⅓ cup salted peanuts

6 to 8 small dried red chiles

1½ teaspoons minced fresh ginger

2 green onions, cut into 1½-inch pieces

1. For marinade, combine 2 teaspoons sherry, 2 teaspoons soy sauce; 2 teaspoons coconut flour and salt in large bowl. Add chicken; stir to coat. Let stand 30 minutes.

2. Combine remaining 3 teaspoons sherry, 3 teaspoons soy sauce, 1½ teaspoons coconut flour, broth and vinegar in small bowl.

3. Heat 1 tablespoon oil in wok or large skillet over medium heat. Add peanuts; stir-fry until lightly toasted. Remove and set aside. Heat remaining 2 tablespoons oil in wok over medium heat. Add chiles; stir-fry until chiles just begin to char, about 1 minute.

4. Increase heat to high. Add chicken mixture; stir-fry 2 minutes. Add ginger; stir-fry about 1 minute or until chicken is cooked through. Stir in peanuts and green onions. Stir sauce mixture; add to wok. Cook and stir until sauce boils and thickens.

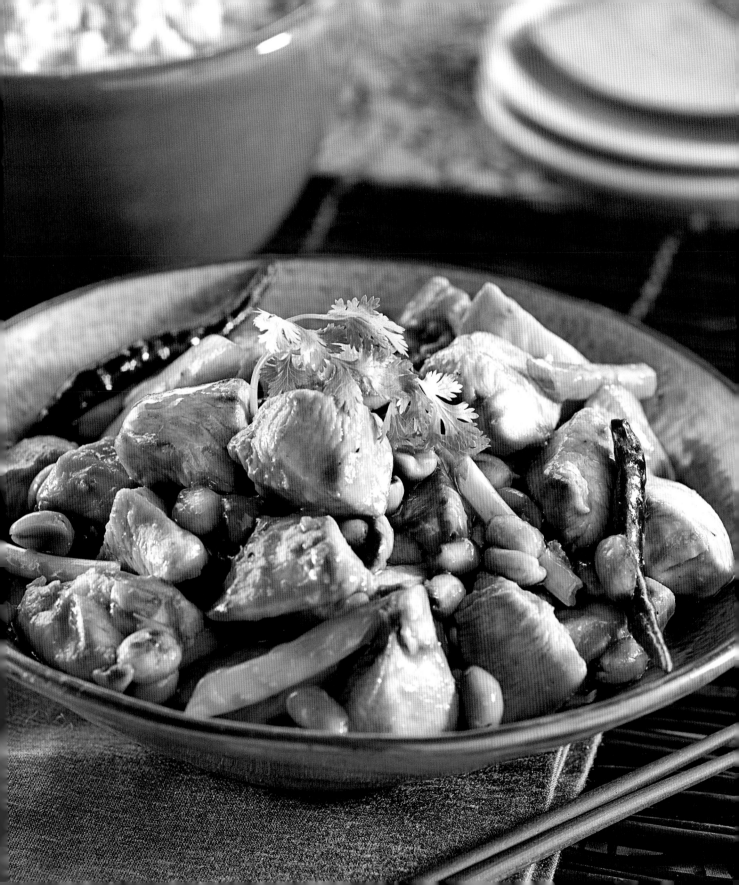

Buffalo Wings

makes 4 servings

PER SERVING

320 calories
25g **total fat**
2g **carbs**
1g **net carbs**
1g **dietary fiber**
20g **protein**

1 cup hot pepper sauce

⅓ cup vegetable oil, plus additional for frying

½ teaspoon ground red pepper

½ teaspoon garlic powder

½ teaspoon Worcestershire sauce

⅛ teaspoon black pepper

1 pound chicken wings, tips discarded, separated at joints

Blue cheese or ranch dressing

Celery sticks

1. Combine hot pepper sauce, ⅓ cup oil, red pepper, garlic powder, Worcestershire sauce and black pepper in small saucepan; cook over medium heat 20 minutes. Remove from heat; pour sauce into large bowl.

2. Heat 3 inches of oil in large saucepan over medium-high heat to 350°F; adjust heat to maintain temperature. Add wings; cook 10 minutes or until crispy. Drain on wire rack set over paper towels.

3. Transfer wings to bowl of sauce; toss to coat. Serve with blue cheese dressing and celery sticks.

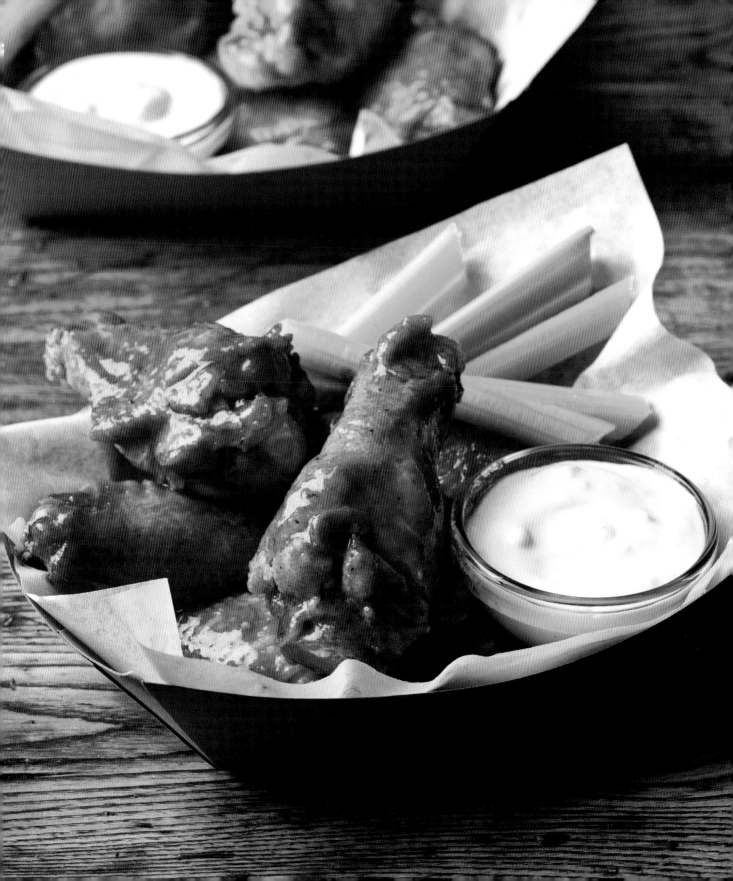

Roasted Chicken with Cabbage

makes 4 servings

⅓ cup olive oil, plus additional for pan

2 tablespoons red wine vinegar

2 cloves garlic, minced

1 teaspoon salt

1 teaspoon onion powder

¼ teaspoon paprika

¼ teaspoon black pepper

8 bone-in, skin-on chicken thighs (about 3 pounds)

1½ medium onions, cut into ½-inch slices (do not separate into rings)

1 small head green cabbage (about 1½ pounds)

Chopped fresh parsley (optional)

1. Preheat oven to 425°F. Brush baking sheet with oil.

2. Whisk ⅓ cup oil, vinegar, garlic, salt, onion powder, paprika and pepper in large bowl until well blended. Remove half of mixture to medium bowl; add chicken and turn to coat.

3. Add onion slices to bowl with oil mixture; turn to coat. Arrange in single layer on prepared baking sheet. Cut cabbage in half through core (do not remove core). Cut each half into 1-inch wedges. Add cabbage to bowl with oil mixture; turn to coat. Arrange cabbage over onions on baking sheet. Place chicken, skin side up, on top of cabbage.

4. Roast 50 to 55 minutes or until chicken is 165°F. Remove chicken to plate; tent with foil to keep warm. Carefully drain liquid from baking sheet. Stir vegetables; roast 10 to 15 minutes or until edges begin to brown and cabbage is crisp-tender. Serve chicken with vegetables. Garnish with parsley.

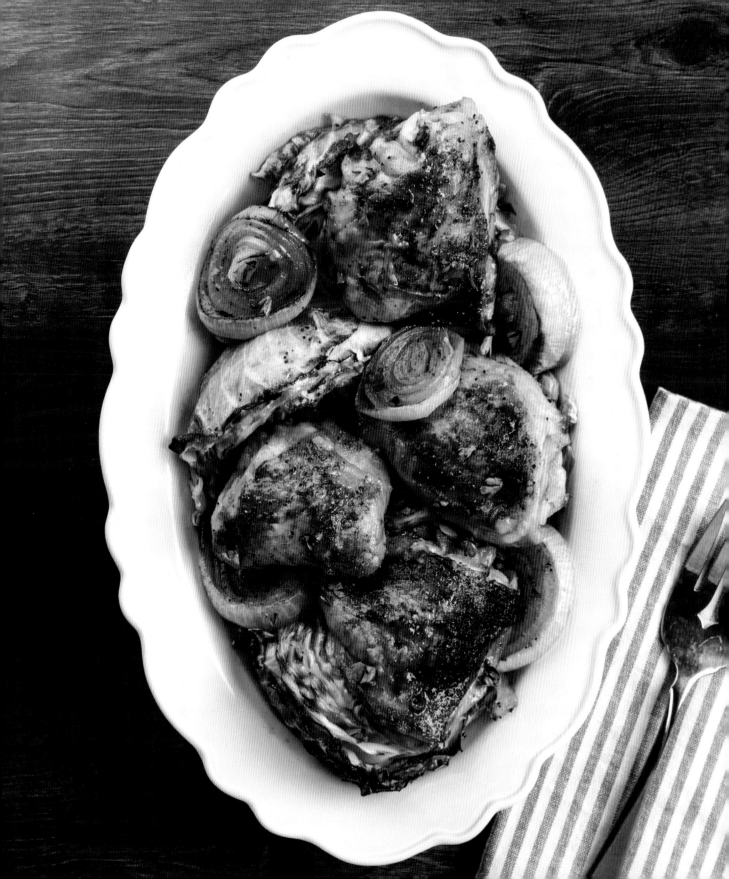

Sheet Pan Chicken and Sausage Supper

makes 6 servings

PER SERVING

430 calories
25g **total fat**
12g **carbs**
10g **net carbs**
2g **dietary fiber**
41g **protein**

⅓ cup olive oil

2 tablespoons balsamic vinegar

1 teaspoon salt

1 teaspoon garlic powder

½ teaspoon black pepper

¼ teaspoon red pepper flakes

3 pounds bone-in chicken thighs and drumsticks

1 pound uncooked sweet Italian sausage (4 to 5 links), cut diagonally into 2-inch pieces

6 small red onions (about 1 pound), each cut into 6 wedges

3½ cups broccoli florets

1. Preheat oven to 425°F. Line baking sheet with foil, if desired.

2. Whisk oil, vinegar, salt, garlic powder, black pepper and red pepper flakes in small bowl until well blended. Combine chicken, sausage and onions on prepared baking sheet. Drizzle with oil mixture; toss until well coated. Spread meat and onions in single layer; turn thighs skin side up.

3. Bake 30 minutes. Add broccoli to baking sheet; stir to coat broccoli with pan juices and turn sausage. Bake 30 minutes or until broccoli is beginning to brown and chicken is cooked through (165°F).

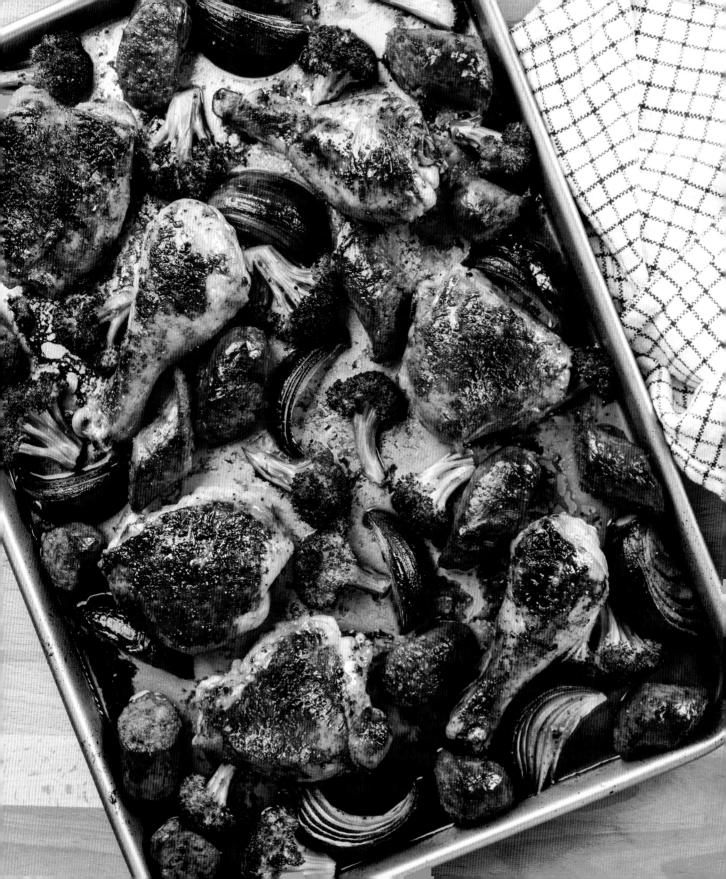

Lemon-Rosemary Roasted Chicken

makes 8 to 10 servings

1 whole chicken (6 to 7 pounds)

1 teaspoon olive oil, divided

1 teaspoon salt, divided

¼ teaspoon black pepper

2 lemons

2½ teaspoons dried rosemary
   or 2 (4-inch) sprigs fresh
   rosemary, leaves chopped,
   divided

2 teaspoons butter, softened

1 large onion, cut into ½-inch
   slices

¾ cup chicken broth

½ teaspoon ground sage

1. Preheat oven to 450°F. Rub chicken with ½ teaspoon oil. Season with ½ teaspoon salt and pepper.

2. Pierce 1 lemon in several places with knife tip or fork; place in chicken cavity. Blend 2 teaspoons rosemary and butter in small bowl. Carefully slide fingers under skin on breast to loosen. Gently smooth butter mixture under skin. Tie legs with kitchen twine, if desired.

3. Place onion slices in center of roasting pan and place chicken on top. Roast 45 minutes, then tent breast with foil. Roast 30 to 40 minutes longer or until internal temperature reaches 165°F. Baste with pan drippings occasionally.

4. Transfer chicken to cutting board; let rest 10 minutes. Pour pan drippings into measuring cup; skim off fat. Squeeze juice from second lemon and add to drippings.

5. Return drippings to roasting pan; add any drippings from chicken. Add remaining ½ teaspoon salt, ½ teaspoon rosemary, broth and sage. Simmer over medium-high heat 2 minutes, scraping up browned bits from bottom of pan. Carve chicken; serve with sauce.

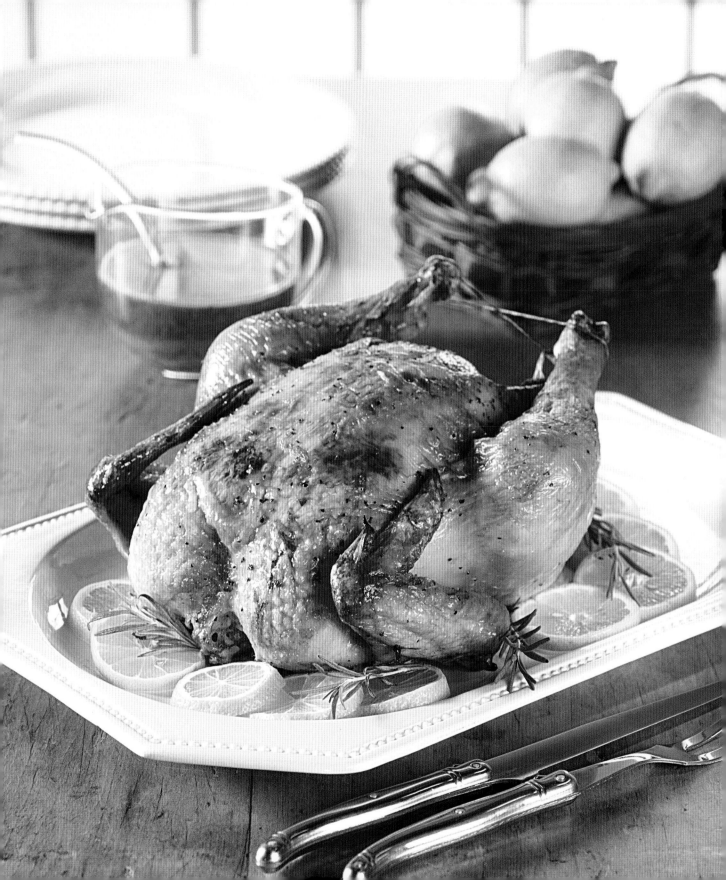

Tangy Chicken Tenders

makes 10 servings

PER SERVING

83 calories
2g **total fat**
5g **carbs**
5g **net carbs**
0g **dietary fiber**
9g **protein**

3 tablespoons Louisiana-style
   hot sauce

½ teaspoon paprika

¼ teaspoon ground red pepper

1 pound chicken tenders

½ cup blue cheese dressing

¼ cup sour cream

2 tablespoons crumbled blue
   cheese

1 medium green or red bell
   pepper, cut into ½-inch slices

1. Preheat oven to 375°F. Combine hot sauce, paprika and ground red pepper in small bowl; brush over chicken. Place chicken in greased 11×7-inch baking dish. Cover; marinate in refrigerator 30 minutes.

2. Uncover; bake about 15 minutes or until chicken is no longer pink in center.

3. Combine blue cheese dressing, sour cream and blue cheese in small serving bowl. Serve with chicken and bell pepper slices.

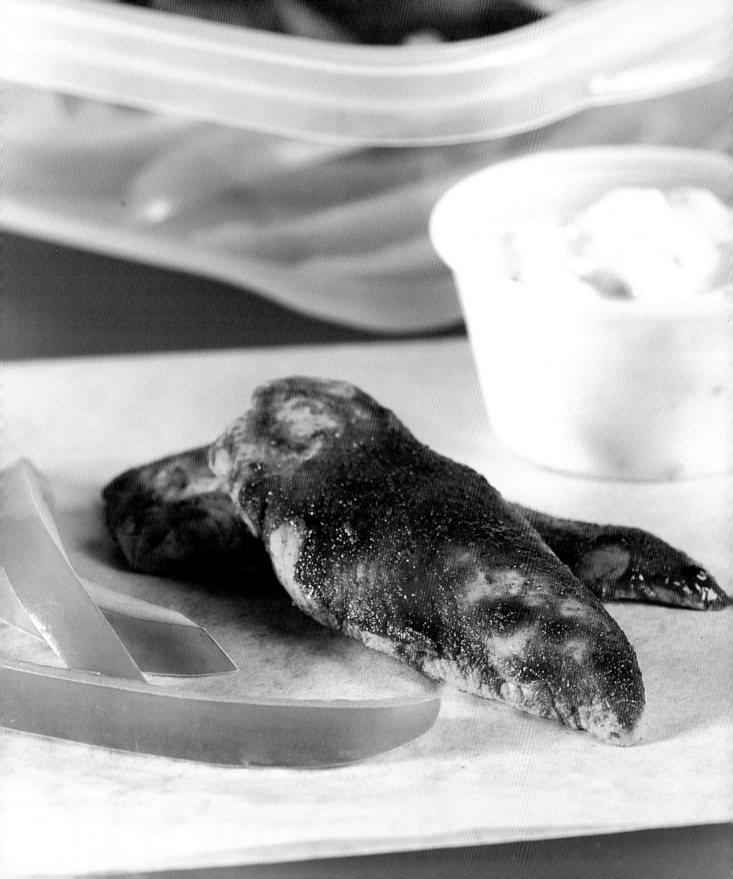

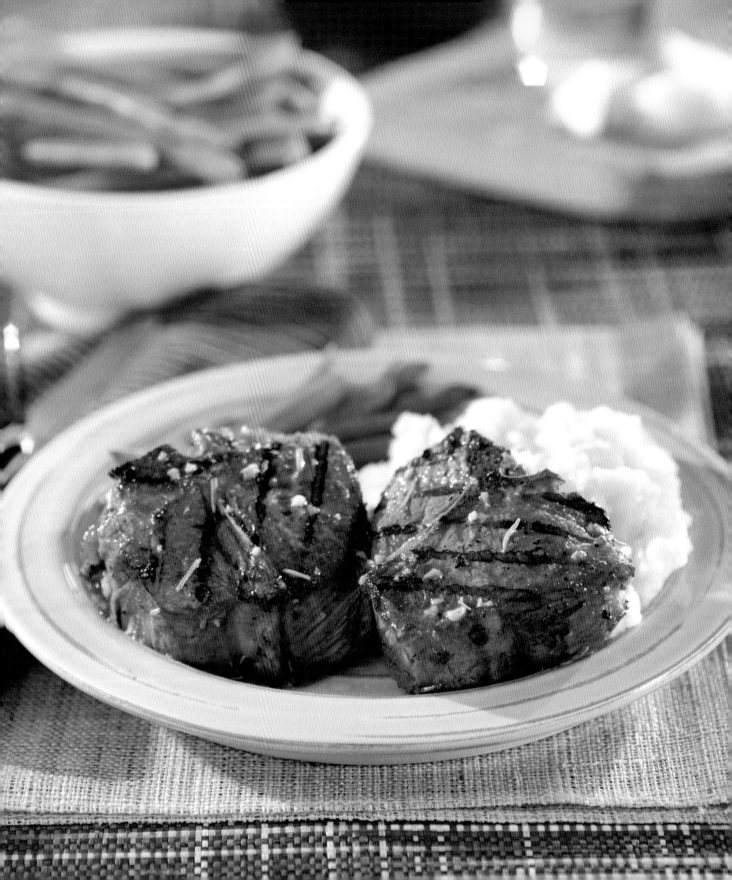

beef, pork *and* lamb

PER SERVING

540 calories
44g total fat
2g carbs
2g net carbs
0g dietary fiber
31g protein

Herbed Lamb Chops

makes 4 servings

⅓ cup olive oil

⅓ cup red wine vinegar

2 tablespoons soy sauce

1 tablespoon lemon juice

3 cloves garlic, minced

1 teaspoon salt

1 teaspoon chopped fresh oregano *or* ¼ teaspoon dried oregano

1 teaspoon dried rosemary

1 teaspoon ground mustard

½ teaspoon white pepper

8 lamb loin chops, 1 inch thick (about 2 pounds)

1. Combine all ingredients except lamb in large resealable food storage bag. Reserve ½ cup marinade in small bowl. Add lamb to remaining marinade. Seal bag; turn to coat. Marinate in refrigerator at least 1 hour.

2. Prepare grill for direct cooking over medium-high heat.

3. Remove lamb from marinade; discard marinade. Grill lamb over medium-high heat 8 minutes or to desired doneness, turning once and basting often with reserved ½ cup marinade. Do not baste during last 5 minutes of cooking. Discard any remaining marinade.

Serving Suggestion: Serve with mashed cauliflower and a steamed green vegetable.

Garlic Beef

makes 4 servings

PER SERVING

214 calories
9g total fat
6g carbs
4g net carbs
2g dietary fiber
27g protein

- 1 teaspoon dark sesame oil
- 1 pound beef eye of round, trimmed, cut into thin strips
- 1 package (10 ounces) frozen chopped broccoli
- 1 tablespoon minced garlic
- 1 tablespoon soy sauce
- ¼ teaspoon black pepper

Heat oil in 12-inch nonstick skillet over high heat. Add beef, broccoli, garlic, soy sauce and pepper. Cook 15 minutes or until beef is done, stirring occasionally.

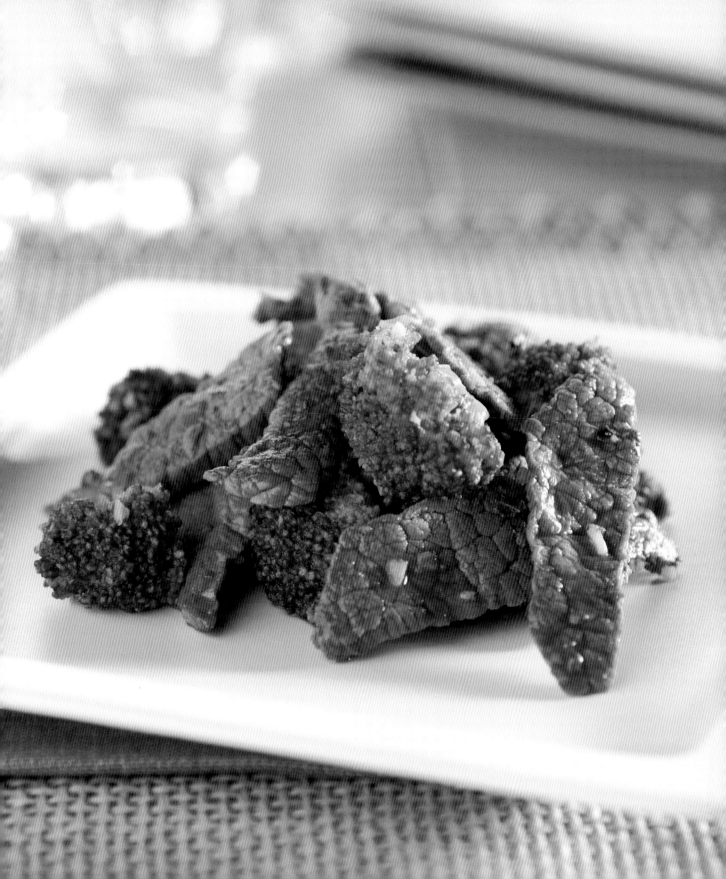

Steaks with Zesty Merlot Sauce

makes 4 servings

PER SERVING

287 calories
17g total fat
4g carbs
3g net carbs
1g dietary fiber
23g protein

½ cup merlot wine

2 tablespoons Worcestershire sauce

1 tablespoon balsamic vinegar

1 teaspoon beef bouillon granules

½ teaspoon dried thyme

2 beef rib-eye steaks (8 ounces each)

2 tablespoons finely chopped fresh parsley

1. Combine wine, Worcestershire sauce, vinegar, bouillon granules and thyme in small bowl; set aside.

2. Heat large nonstick skillet over high heat until hot. Add steaks; cook 3 minutes on each side. Turn steaks again and cook 3 to 6 minutes longer over medium heat or until desired doneness.

3. Cut steaks in half; arrange on serving platter. Tent with foil; keep warm.

4. Add wine mixture to skillet; bring to a boil. Cook and stir 1 minute, scraping up any brown bits from bottom of skillet. Spoon over steaks. Sprinkle with parsley; serve immediately.

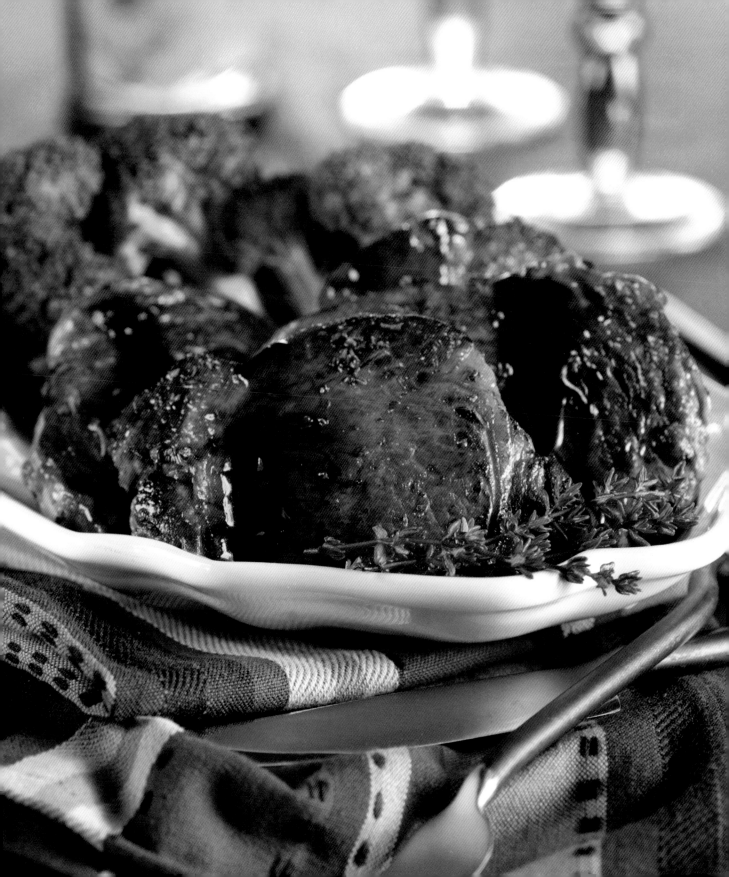

Blue Cheese-Stuffed Sirloin Patties

makes 4 servings

1½ pounds ground sirloin

½ **cup (2 ounces) shredded sharp Cheddar cheese**

¼ **cup crumbled blue cheese**

¼ **cup finely chopped fresh parsley**

2 **teaspoons Dijon mustard**

1 **teaspoon Worcestershire sauce**

1 **clove garlic, minced**

¼ **teaspoon salt**

2 **teaspoons olive oil**

1 **medium red bell pepper, cut into thin strips**

1. Shape beef into 8 patties, about 4 inches in diameter and ¼ inch thick.

2. Combine cheeses, parsley, mustard, Worcestershire sauce, garlic and ¼ teaspoon salt in small bowl; toss gently.

3. Mound one fourth of cheese mixture on each of 4 patties (about 3 tablespoons per patty). Top with remaining 4 patties; pinch edges of patties to seal completely.

4. Heat oil in large skillet over medium-high heat. Add bell pepper; cook and stir 5 minutes or until edges of peppers begin to brown. Season with salt. Transfer to plate; keep warm.

5. Add beef patties to same skillet; cook 5 minutes. Turn patties; top with bell peppers. Cook 4 minutes or until medium (160°F) or to desired doneness.

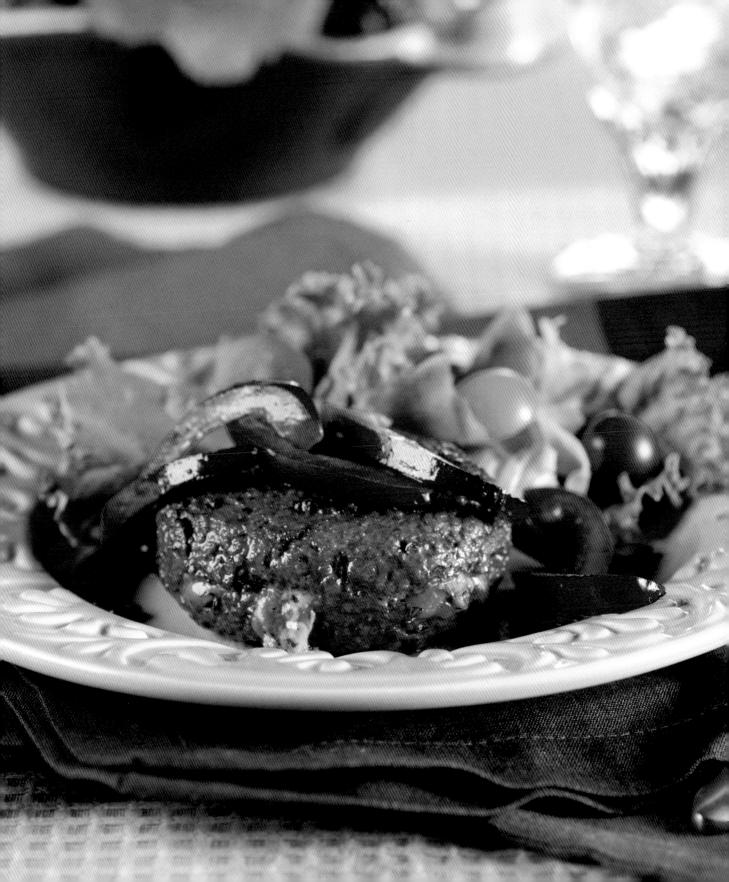

Greek-Style Braised Lamb Chops

makes 4 servings

1 teaspoon Greek seasoning

4 lamb shoulder chops (about 2½ pounds)

3 tablespoons olive oil

1 large onion, halved and sliced

1½ cups beef broth

3 plum tomatoes, each cut into 6 wedges

½ cup pitted kalamata olives

1 tablespoon chopped fresh parsley

1. Rub Greek seasoning into chops.

2. Heat oil in large skillet over medium-high heat. Working in 2 batches, add chops and brown on all sides. Transfer chops to large plate.

3. Add onion to skillet; cook and stir 3 to 5 minutes or until softened. Pour in broth. Bring to a boil over high heat, scraping up browned bits from bottom of skillet. Reduce heat to low; add chops, tomatoes and olives. Cover and simmer over low heat 1 hour or until meat is tender.

4. Transfer chops and vegetables to serving platter using slotted spoon; tent with foil to keep warm. Bring remaining liquid to a boil over high heat; cook until slightly thickened. Reduce to about 1 cup. Pour sauce over chops and vegetables; sprinkle with parsley.

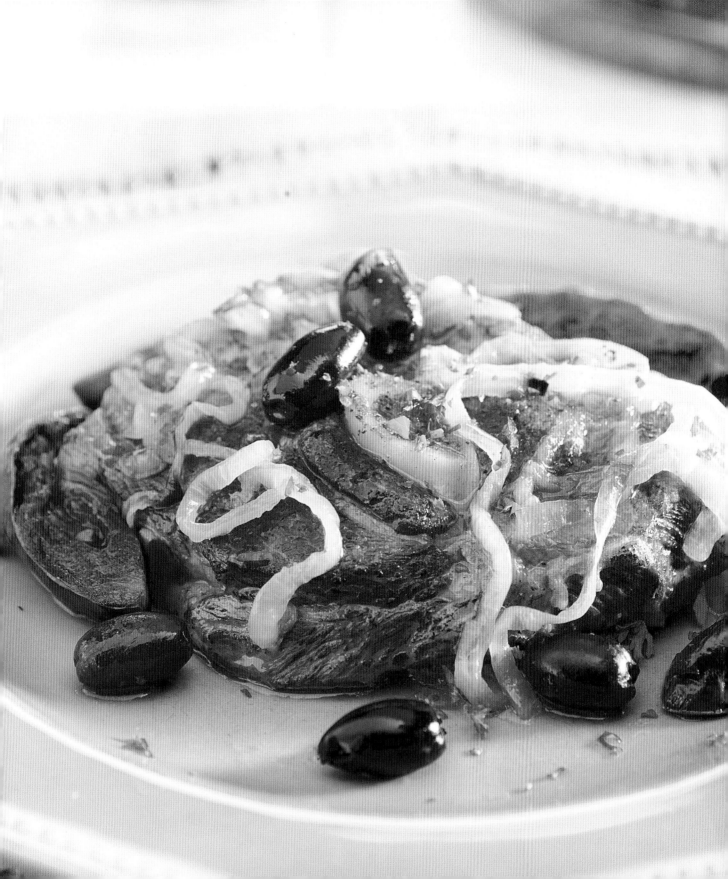

Grilled Steak and Asparagus Salad

makes 4 servings

PER SERVING

189 calories
8g total fat
10g carbs
7g net carbs
3g dietary fiber
20g protein

1 boneless top sirloin steak (10 ounces and about 1-inch thick), trimmed of visible fat

1 teaspoon garlic-herb seasoning blend

1 pound fresh asparagus, trimmed

1 teaspoon canola oil

6 cups spring salad greens

½ cup chopped green onions

¼ cup champagne vinaigrette or balsamic vinaigrette

4 teaspoons crumbled blue cheese

1. Prepare grill for direct cooking. Season steak with seasoning blend. Grill steak, covered, over medium heat about 8 to 10 minutes, turning once, until steak is still pink in center. Remove from grill. Cover loosely with foil to keep warm.

2. Place asparagus in grill basket; drizzle with oil and roll to coat. Grill over medium heat 3 to 5 minutes or until crisp-tender, shaking basket once or twice. Remove from grill.

3. Meanwhile, toss salad greens, green onions and vinaigrette in large bowl. Divide salad among 4 plates. Thinly slice steak across the grain. Divide among salad plates. Top each salad with asparagus and sprinkle with blue cheese.

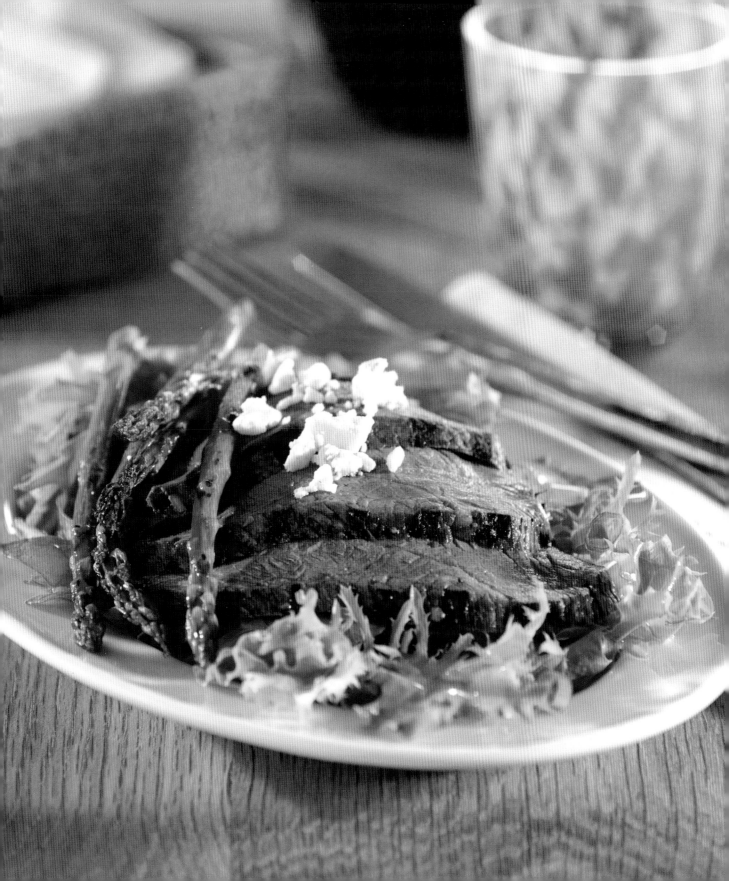

Oregano Beef Kabobs

makes 4 servings

PER SERVING

163 calories
4g **total fat**
8g **carbs**
7g **net carbs**
1g **dietary fiber**
22g **protein**

¼ cup dry red wine

¼ cup finely chopped fresh parsley

2 tablespoons Worcestershire sauce

1 tablespoon soy sauce

1 teaspoon dried oregano

3 cloves garlic, minced

½ teaspoon salt

½ teaspoon black pepper

12 ounces boneless beef top sirloin steak, cut into 16 (1-inch) pieces

16 whole mushrooms (about 8 ounces total)

1 medium red onion, cut in eighths and layers separated

1. Combine wine, parsley, Worcestershire sauce, soy sauce, oregano, garlic, salt and pepper in small bowl; stir until well blended. Place steak, mushrooms and onion in resealable food storage bag. Add wine mixture; seal bag and turn to coat. Marinate in refrigerator 1 hour, turning frequently.

2. Soak 4 (12-inch) or 8 (6-inch) bamboo skewers in water for 20 minutes to prevent burning.

3. Preheat broiler. Alternate beef, mushrooms and 2 layers of onion on skewers.

4. Coat broiler rack with nonstick cooking spray. Arrange skewers on broiler rack; brush with marinade. Broil 4 to 6 inches from heat source 8 to 10 minutes, turning occasionally.

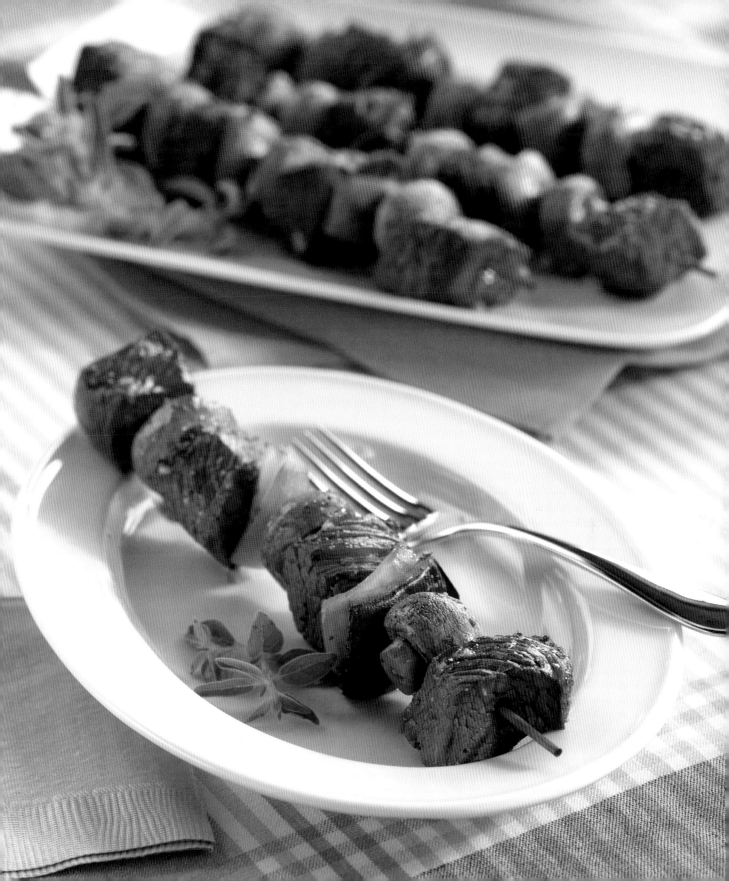

Spicy Asian Pork Bundles

makes 20 bundles

PER SERVING

100 calories
4g total fat
1g carbs
1g net carbs
0g dietary fiber
16g protein

1 boneless pork sirloin roast
(about 3 pounds)

½ cup tamari or other soy sauce

1 tablespoon chile garlic sauce or
chile paste

2 teaspoons minced fresh ginger

2 tablespoons water

1 tablespoon coconut flour

2 teaspoons dark sesame oil

20 large lettuce leaves

Slow Cooker Directions

1. Cut roast into 2- to 3-inch chunks. Combine pork, tamari sauce, chile garlic sauce and ginger in slow cooker; mix well. Cover; cook on LOW 8 to 10 hours.

2. Remove pork from cooking liquid; cool slightly. Trim and discard excess fat. Shred pork using two forks. Let liquid stand 5 minutes to allow fat to rise. Skim off fat.

3. Blend water, coconut flour and sesame oil in small bowl until smooth; stir into slow cooker. Cook, uncovered, on HIGH until thickened. Add shredded meat to slow cooker; mix well. Cover; cook on HIGH 15 to 30 minutes or until hot. Place ¼ cup pork filling into large lettuce leaves. Wrap to enclose.

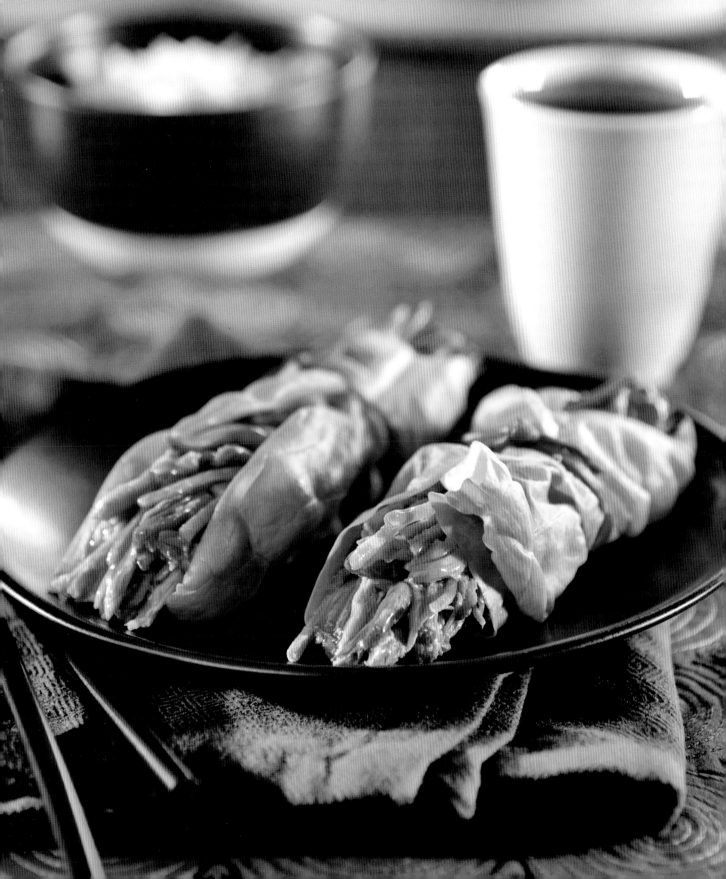

Flank Steak
with Italian Salsa

makes 6 servings

PER SERVING

191 calories
11g total fat
4g carbs
3g net carbs
1g dietary fiber
18g protein

2 tablespoons olive oil

2 teaspoons balsamic vinegar

1 lean flank steak (1½ pounds)

1 tablespoon minced garlic

¾ teaspoon salt, divided

¾ teaspoon black pepper, divided

1 cup diced plum tomatoes

⅓ cup chopped pitted kalamata
   olives

2 tablespoons chopped fresh
   basil

1. Whisk oil and vinegar in medium bowl until well blended. Place steak in shallow dish. Spread garlic over steak; sprinkle with ½ teaspoon salt and ½ teaspoon pepper. Spoon 2 tablespoons oil mixture over steak. Marinate in refrigerator at least 20 minutes or up to 2 hours.

2. Add tomatoes, olives, basil, remaining ¼ teaspoon salt and ¼ teaspoon pepper to remaining 2 teaspoons vinegar mixture in bowl; mix well.

3. Prepare grill for direct cooking or preheat broiler. Remove steak from marinade; discard marinade. (Leave garlic on steak.)

4. Grill steak over medium-high heat 5 to 6 minutes per side for medium rare. Remove to cutting board; tent with foil and let stand 5 minutes. Cut steak diagonally across the grain into thin slices. Serve with tomato mixture.

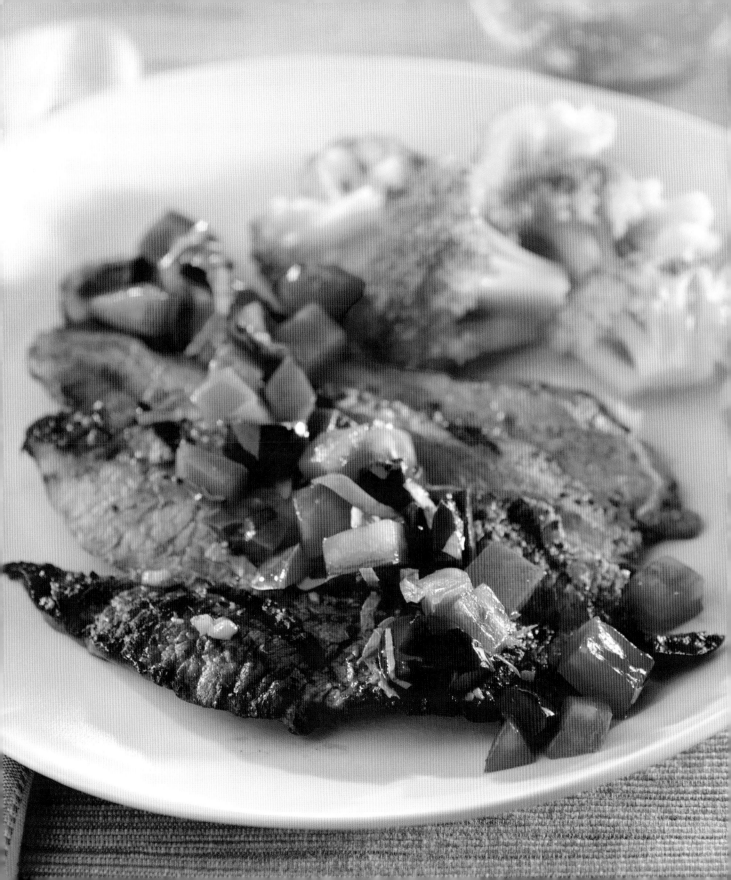

Thai Grilled Beef Salad

makes 4 servings

PER SERVING

200 calories
6g total fat
7g carbs
4g net carbs
3g dietary fiber
26g protein

3 tablespoons Thai seasoning blend, divided

1 beef flank steak (about 1 pound)

2 tablespoons chopped fresh cilantro

2 tablespoons chopped fresh basil

2 red Thai peppers *or* 1 red jalapeño pepper, seeded and sliced into thin slivers

1 tablespoon finely chopped lemongrass

1 tablespoon minced red onion

1 clove garlic, minced

Juice of 1 lime

1 tablespoon fish sauce

1 large carrot, grated

1 cucumber, chopped

4 cups assorted salad greens

1. Prepare grill for direct grilling.

2. Sprinkle 1 tablespoon Thai seasoning over beef; turn to coat. Cover and let stand 15 minutes. Place steak on grid over medium heat. Grill, uncovered, 17 to 21 minutes for medium rare to medium or until desired doneness, turning once. Cool 10 minutes.

3. Meanwhile, combine remaining 2 tablespoons Thai seasoning, cilantro, basil, chile peppers, lemongrass, onion, garlic, lime juice and fish sauce in medium bowl; mix well.

4. Thinly slice beef across grain. Add beef, carrot and cucumber to dressing; toss to coat. Arrange on bed of greens.

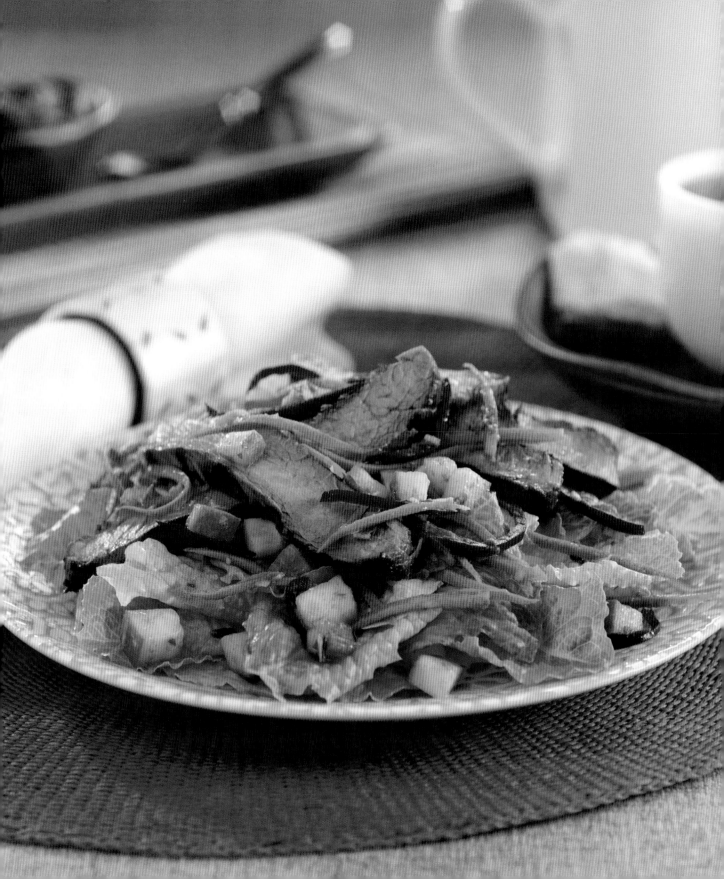

Pork Chops Bolognese

makes 4 servings

PER SERVING

520 calories
37g total fat
1g carbs
1g net carbs
0g dietary fiber
44g protein

- 4 (¾-inch-thick) bone-in rib pork chops (1 pound total)
- 4 slices prosciutto (4 ounces)
- 4 slices fontina cheese (4 ounces)
- 2 teaspoons chopped fresh rosemary leaves
- 1 teaspoon chopped fresh sage (optional)
- 2 cloves garlic, minced
  Salt and black pepper
- 2 to 3 tablespoons olive oil

1. Preheat oven to 350°F. Split chops horizontally in half, stopping at bone. Open each chop and arrange 1 slice of prosciutto, folding to fit. Top prosciutto with cheese; trim to fit chops.

2. Sprinkle outside of chops with rosemary, sage, if desired, garlic, salt and pepper. Heat 2 tablespoons oil over medium-high heat in ovenproof skillet large enough to hold chops in single layer. Brown chops 1 to 2 minutes on each side, adding additional oil if needed.

3. Transfer skillet to oven and bake 6 to 10 minutes or until chops are cooked through (160°F).

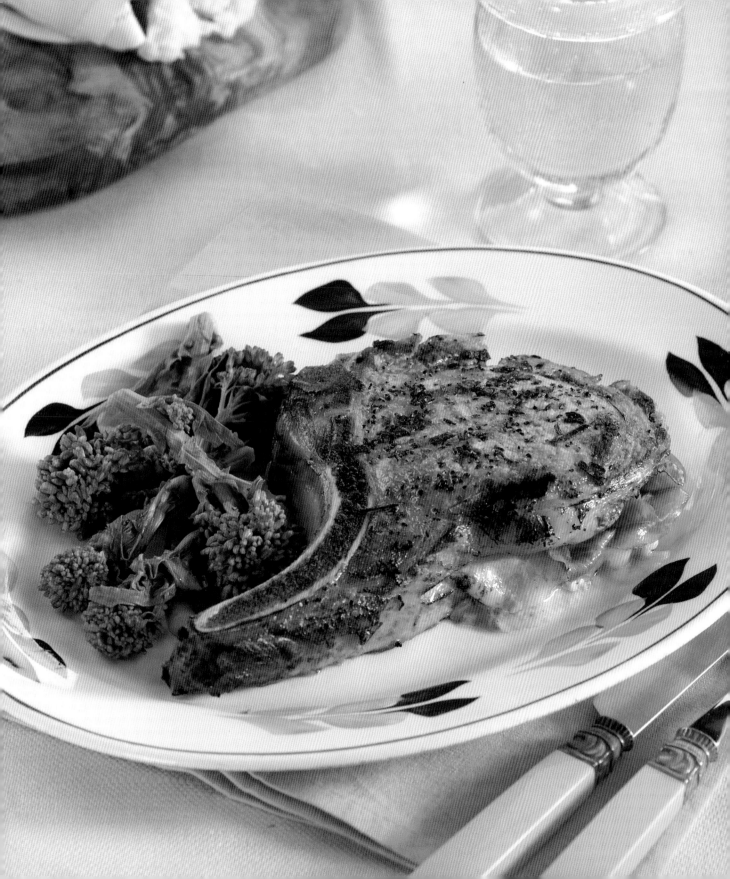

Meatballs and Ricotta

makes 7 servings (21 meatballs)

PER SERVING

643 calories
43g **total fat**
22g **carbs**
16g **net carbs**
6g **dietary fiber**
38g **protein**

Meatballs

- 2 tablespoons olive oil
- ½ cup almond flour
- ½ cup milk
- 1 cup minced yellow onion
- 2 green onions, finely chopped
- ½ cup grated Romano cheese
- 2 eggs, beaten
- ¼ cup minced fresh parsley
- ¼ cup minced fresh basil
- 2 cloves garlic, minced
- 2 teaspoons salt
- ¼ teaspoon black pepper
- 1 pound ground beef
- 1 pound ground pork

Sauce

- 2 tablespoons olive oil
- 2 tablespoons butter
- 1 cup chopped yellow onion
- 1 clove garlic, minced
- 1 can (28 ounces) whole Italian plum tomatoes, coarsely chopped, juice reserved
- 1 can (28 ounces) crushed tomatoes
- 1 teaspoon salt
- ¼ teaspoon black pepper
- ¼ cup finely chopped fresh basil
- 1 cup ricotta cheese

1. Preheat oven to 375°F. Brush 2 tablespoons oil over large rimmed baking sheet.

2. Combine almond flour and milk in large bowl; mix well. Add minced yellow onion, green onions, Romano, eggs, parsley, ¼ cup basil, 2 cloves garlic, 2 teaspoons salt and ¼ teaspoon black pepper; mix well. Add beef and pork; mix gently but thoroughly until blended. Shape mixture by ¼ cupfuls into balls. Place meatballs on prepared baking sheet; turn to coat with oil.

3. Bake about 20 minutes or until meatballs are cooked through (165°F).

4. Meanwhile for sauce, heat 2 tablespoons oil and butter in large saucepan over medium heat until butter is melted. Add chopped yellow onion; cook 8 minutes or until tender and lightly browned, stirring frequently. Add 1 clove garlic; cook and stir 1 minute or until fragrant. Add plum tomatoes with juice, crushed tomatoes, 1 teaspoon salt and ¼ teaspoon black pepper; bring to a simmer. Reduce heat to medium-low; cook 20 minutes, stirring occasionally.

5. Stir ¼ cup basil into sauce. Add meatballs; cook 10 minutes, stirring occasionally. Transfer meatballs and sauce to serving dish; dollop tablespoonfuls of ricotta between meatballs.

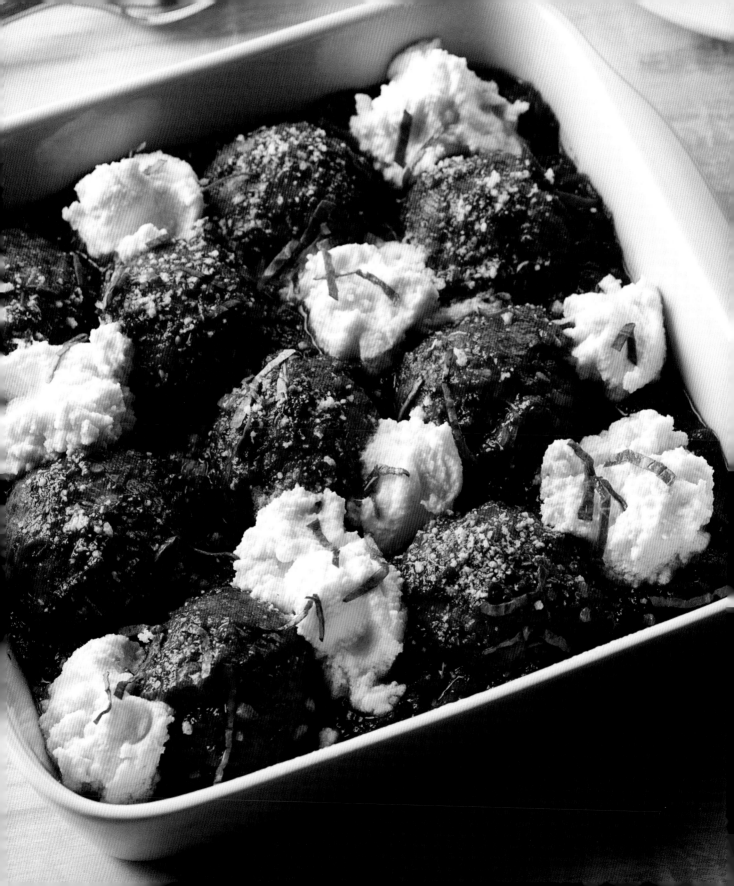

Mediterranean Steak Salad

makes 4 servings

PER SERVING

580 calories
40g **total fat**
9g **carbs**
5g **net carbs**
2g **dietary fiber**
49g **protein**

Steak

- 4 sirloin steaks (about 8 ounces each)
- 2 tablespoons olive oil, divided
- 2 teaspoons salt
- 2 teaspoons dried oregano
- 2 teaspoons paprika
- 1 teaspoon black pepper
- 2 cloves garlic, minced

Salad and Dressing

- ⅓ cup olive oil
- 3 tablespoons red wine vinegar
- 1 clove garlic, minced
- ¾ teaspoon dried oregano
- ¾ teaspoon salt
- ¼ teaspoon black pepper
- 4 cups assorted mixed greens
- 2 medium tomatoes, cut into wedges
- ½ red onion, thinly sliced
- ½ cup pitted kalamata olives
- 4 ounces feta cheese, cut into cubes

1. Combine 2 tablespoons oil, 2 teaspoons salt, 2 teaspoons dried oregano, paprika, 1 teaspoon black pepper and 1 clove garlic in large bowl. Add steak; toss until well coated.

2. Oil grid. Prepare grill for direct cooking. Cook steak, covered, over medium-high heat about 6 minutes per side for medium.

3. For dressing, whisk ⅓ cup oil, vinegar, 1 clove garlic, ¾ teaspoon oregano, ¾ teaspoons salt and ¼ teaspoon pepper in medium bowl.

4. Divide greens among 4 plates. Top with tomatoes, onion, cheese, olives and steak. Drizzle with dressing.

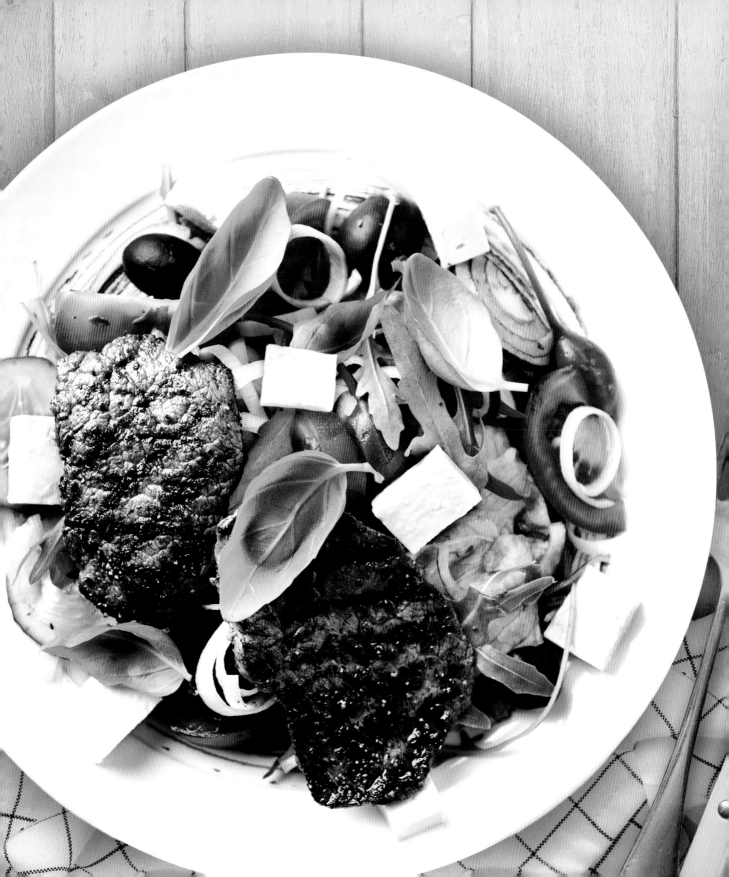

Pork and Peppers Mexican-Style

makes 4 servings

2 tablespoons olive oil

½ cup chopped green onions

12 ounces lean pork, cut into ¼-inch pieces

1 *each* red, yellow and green bell peppers, diced (about 2 cups)

1 teaspoon minced garlic

Salt and black pepper

1 cup sliced mushrooms

1 teaspoon ground cumin

1 teaspoon chili powder

½ teaspoon chipotle chili powder (optional)

¼ cup (1 ounce) shredded Cheddar cheese

¼ cup sour cream

1. Heat oil in large skillet over medium-high heat. Add green onions; cook and stir 2 minutes. Add pork; cook and stir 5 minutes or until browned. Add bell peppers and garlic; cook and stir 5 minutes or until bell peppers begin to soften.

2. Season mixture with salt and black pepper. Add mushrooms, cumin, chili powder and chipotle chili powder, if desired. Cook and stir 10 to 15 minutes until pork is cooked through and vegetables are tender. Serve with shredded cheese and sour cream.

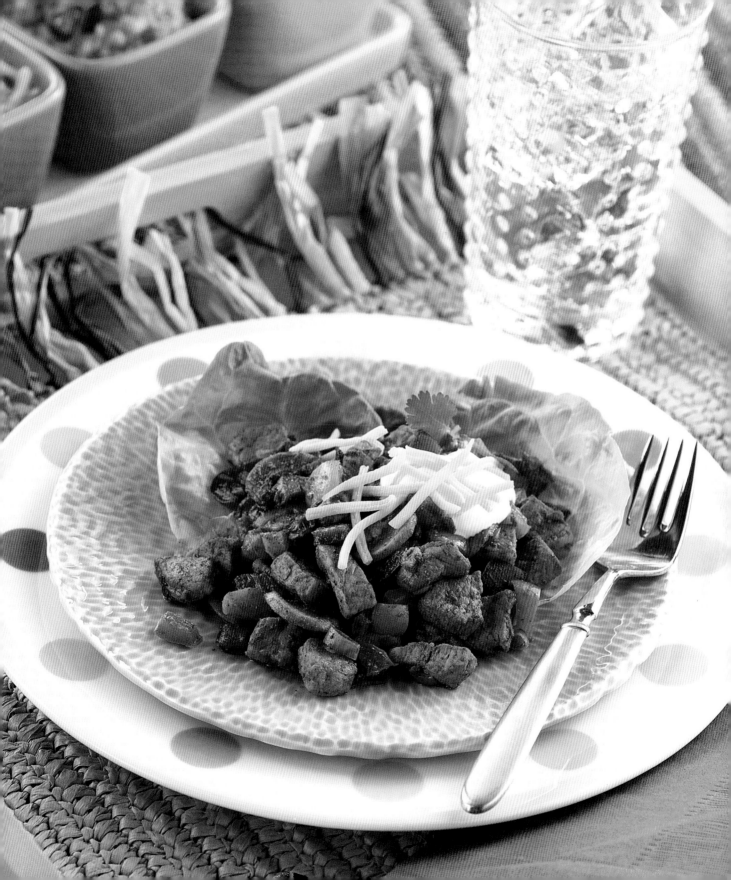

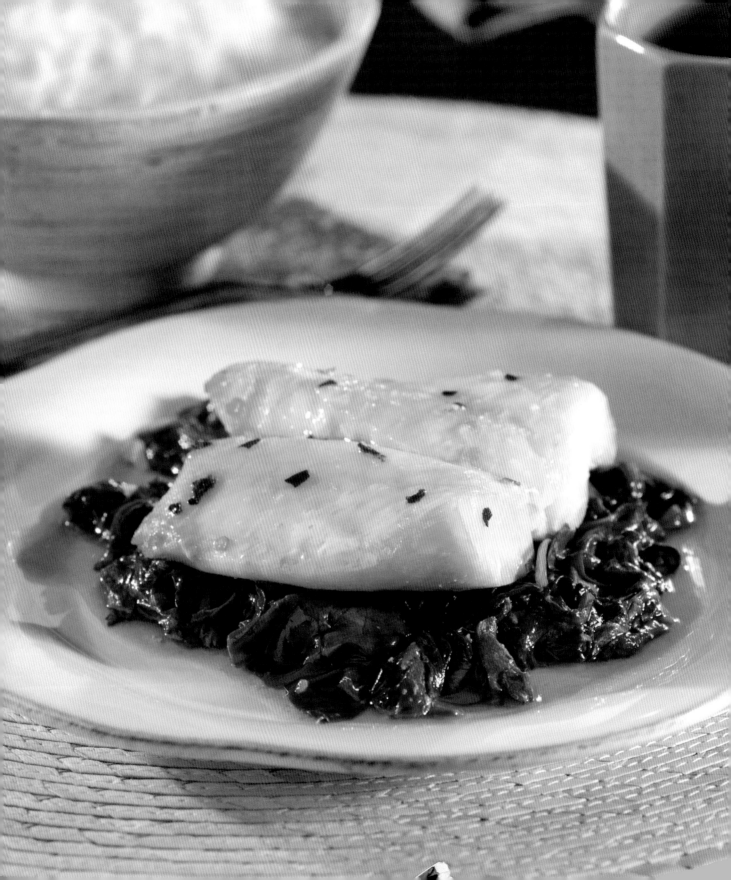

fish and seafood

Shanghai Fish Packets

makes 4 servings

4 tilapia, sole or halibut fillets (6 ounces each)

¼ cup mirin* or Rhine wine

3 tablespoons soy sauce

1 tablespoon dark sesame oil

1½ teaspoons grated fresh ginger

¼ teaspoon red pepper flakes

1 tablespoon peanut or olive oil

1 clove garlic, minced

1 package (10 ounces) fresh spinach leaves, stems removed

Mirin is a Japanese sweet wine available in Japanese markets and the gourmet section of large supermarkets.

1. Prepare grill for direct cooking.

2. Place fish in single layer in large shallow dish. Combine mirin, soy sauce, sesame oil, ginger and red pepper flakes in small bowl; pour over fish. Cover and marinate in refrigerator 20 minutes.

3. Heat peanut oil in large skillet over medium heat. Add garlic; cook and stir 1 minute. Add spinach; cook and stir about 3 minutes until wilted.

4. Place spinach mixture in center of four 12-inch squares of heavy-duty foil. Remove fish from marinade; reserve marinade. Place 1 fish fillet over each mound of spinach; drizzle with reserved marinade. Wrap in foil to create packet, leaving head space for heat circulation.

5. Grill packets, covered, over medium heat 15 to 18 minutes or until fish begins to flake when tested with fork.*

Or place packets on sheet pan and bake at 350°F for 15 minutes or until fish begins to flake when tested with fork.

135

Baked Fish with Thai Pesto

makes 6 servings

PER SERVING

530 **calories**
43g **total fat**
4g **carbs**
2g **net carbs**
2g **dietary fiber**
33g **protein**

- 1 to 2 jalapeño peppers, seeded and coarsely chopped
- 1 lemon
- 4 green onions, thinly sliced
- 2 tablespoons chopped fresh ginger
- 3 cloves garlic, minced
- 1½ cups lightly packed fresh basil leaves
- 1 cup lightly packed fresh cilantro leaves
- ¼ cup lightly packed fresh mint leaves
- ¼ cup unsalted roasted peanuts
- 2 tablespoons unsweetened shredded coconut
- ½ cup peanut oil
- 2 pounds boneless fish fillets (such as salmon, halibut, cod or orange roughy)

1. Place jalapeños in blender or food processor.

2. Grate peel of lemon. Juice lemon to measure 2 tablespoons. Add peel and juice to blender.

3. Add green onions, ginger, garlic, basil, cilantro, mint, peanuts and coconut to blender; blend until finely chopped. With motor running, drizzle in oil in thin steady stream.

4. Preheat oven to 375°F. Rinse fish and pat dry with paper towels. Place fillets on lightly oiled baking sheet. Spread layer of pesto over each fillet.

5. Bake 10 minutes or until fish begins to flake when tested with fork and is just opaque in center. Transfer fish to serving platter with wide spatula.

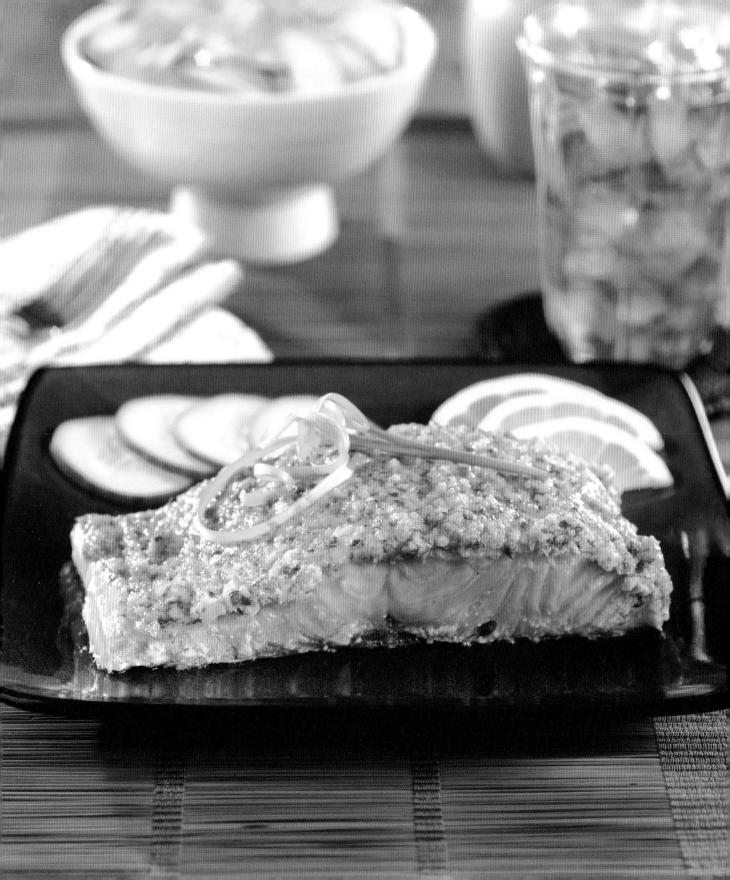

Grilled Scallops and Vegetables with Cilantro Sauce

makes 4 servings

PER SERVING

194 calories
7g **total fat**
11g **carbs**
8g **net carbs**
3g **dietary fiber**
23g **protein**

- 1 teaspoon hot chili oil
- 1 teaspoon dark sesame oil
- 1 green onion, chopped
- 1 tablespoon finely chopped fresh ginger
- 1 cup chicken broth
- 1 cup chopped fresh cilantro
- 1 pound raw or thawed frozen sea scallops
- 2 medium zucchini, cut into ½-inch slices
- 2 medium yellow squash, cut into ½-inch slices
- 1 medium yellow onion, cut into wedges
- 8 large mushrooms

1. Spray grid with nonstick cooking spray. Prepare grill for direct cooking. If using wooden skewers, soak in water 25 to 30 minutes before using to prevent skewers from burning.

2. Heat chili oil and sesame oil in small saucepan over medium-low heat. Add green onion; cook and stir about 15 seconds or just until fragrant. Add ginger; cook and stir 1 minute. Stir in broth; bring to a boil. Cook until liquid is reduced by half; cool slightly. Pour into blender or food processor; add cilantro and blend until smooth. (Or add cilantro to saucepan and use hand-held immersion blender to blend mixture until smooth.)

3. Thread scallops and vegetables onto four 12-inch skewers.

4. Grill over medium-high heat about 8 minutes per side or until scallops turn opaque. Serve hot with cilantro sauce.

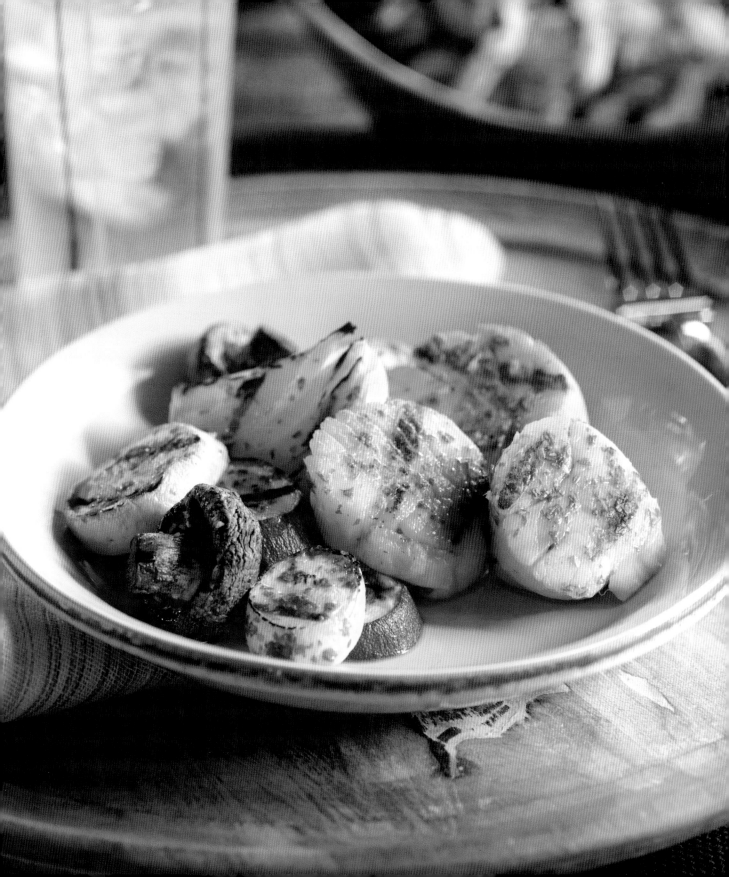

Spicy Crabmeat Frittata

makes 4 servings

1 can (about 6 ounces) lump white crabmeat, drained

6 eggs

¼ teaspoon salt

¼ teaspoon black pepper

¼ teaspoon hot pepper sauce

1 tablespoon olive oil

1 green bell pepper, finely chopped

2 cloves garlic, minced

1 plum tomato, seeded and finely chopped

1. Preheat broiler. Pick out and discard any shell or cartilage from crabmeat; break up large pieces of crabmeat.

2. Beat eggs in medium bowl. Add crabmeat, salt, black pepper and hot pepper sauce; mix well.

3. Heat oil in large ovenproof skillet over medium-high heat. Add bell pepper and garlic; cook and stir 3 minutes or until tender. Add tomato; cook and stir 1 minute. Stir in egg mixture; cook over medium-low heat 7 minutes or until eggs begin to set around edges.

4. Transfer skillet to broiler. Broil 4 inches from heat source 1 to 2 minutes or until frittata is golden brown and center is set.

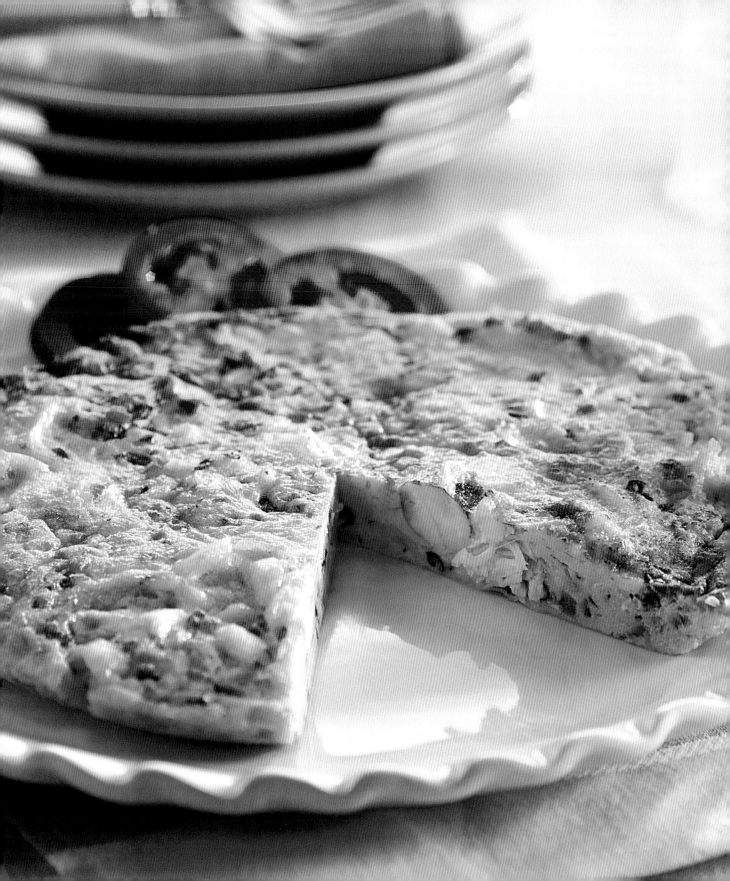

Skillet-Grilled Catfish and Creole Salsa

makes 4 servings

Creole Salsa

- 1 cup finely chopped tomatoes
- ⅓ cup finely chopped green bell pepper
- ¼ cup finely chopped celery
- ¼ cup minced green onions
- 2 tablespoons minced fresh parsley
- 2 teaspoons cider vinegar
- ¾ teaspoon dried thyme
- ¼ teaspoon salt
- ¼ to ½ teaspoon hot pepper sauce

Catfish

- 4 catfish fillets (4 ounces each), rinsed and patted dry
- 1 teaspoon steak seasoning or blackened seasoning
- ¼ teaspoon salt
- 4 lemon wedges

1. Combine tomatoes, bell pepper, celery, green onions, parsley, vinegar, thyme, ¼ teaspoon salt and hot pepper sauce in medium bowl. Set aside.

2. Sprinkle one side of each fillet evenly with steak seasoning and ¼ teaspoon salt.

3. Spray large nonstick skillet over medium-high heat. Add fish seasoned side down; cook 3 minutes. Turn and cook 3 minutes or until fish is opaque in center. Squeeze lemon wedges over fish. Serve with salsa.

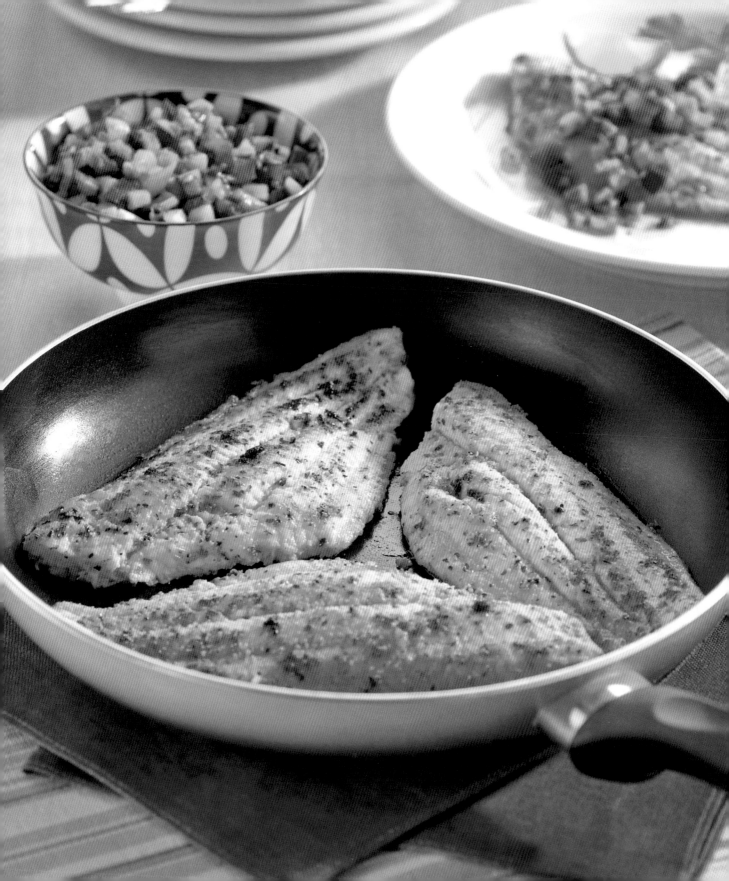

Szechuan Tuna Steaks

makes 4 servings

PER SERVING

284 calories
11g total fat
2g carbs
1g net carbs
1g dietary fiber
40g protein

- **4** tuna steaks (6 ounces each), cut 1 inch thick
- **¼** cup dry sherry or sake
- **¼** cup soy sauce
- **1** tablespoon dark sesame oil
- **1** teaspoon hot chili oil *or* ¼ teaspoon red pepper flakes
- **1** clove garlic, minced
- **3** tablespoons chopped fresh cilantro (optional)

1. Place tuna in single layer in large shallow glass dish. Combine sherry, soy sauce, sesame oil, hot chili oil and garlic in small bowl. Reserve ¼ cup soy sauce mixture at room temperature. Pour remaining soy sauce mixture over fish; cover and marinate in refrigerator 40 minutes, turning once.

2. Spray grid with nonstick cooking spray. Prepare grill for direct cooking. Drain fish, discarding marinade.

3. Grill fish, uncovered, over medium-high heat 6 minutes or until tuna is seared but still feels somewhat soft in center,* turning halfway through grilling time. Remove to to cutting board. Cut into thin slices; drizzle with reserved soy sauce mixture. Garnish with cilantro.

Tuna becomes dry and tough if overcooked. Cook to medium doneness for best results.

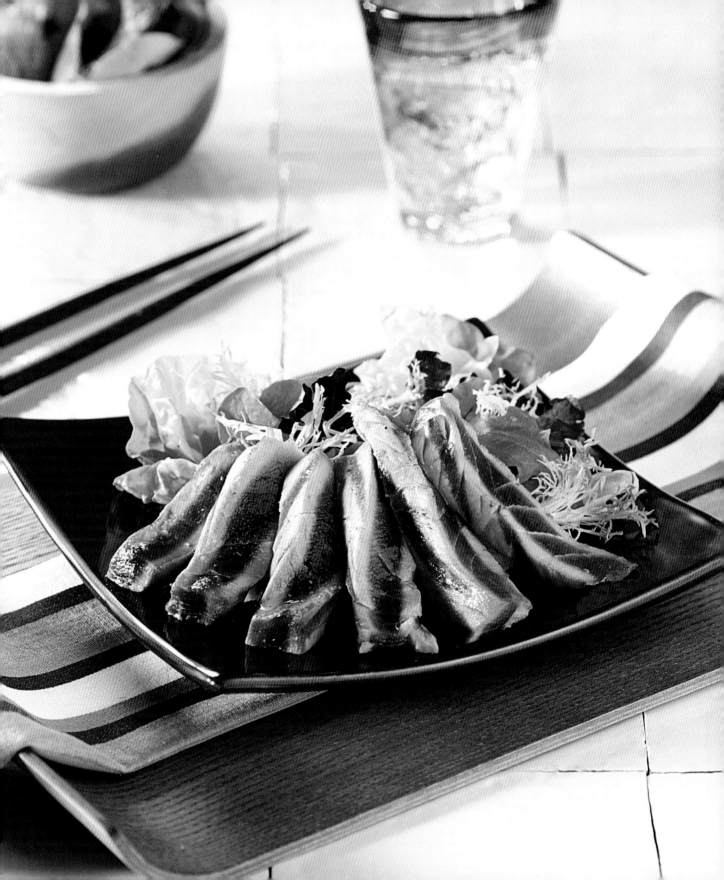

Shrimp Rémoulade Salad

makes 4 servings

PER SERVING

177 **calories**
5g **total fat**
10g **carbs**
6g **net carbs**
4g **dietary fiber**
21g **protein**

12 ounces cooked shrimp, peeled and deveined

2 cups shredded red cabbage

2 stalks celery, finely sliced

½ cup sliced green onions

3 tablespoons sugar-free ketchup

2 tablespoons prepared horseradish

1½ tablespoons white wine vinegar

1 tablespoon olive oil

1 tablespoon Dijon mustard

2 cloves garlic, minced

¼ teaspoon salt

1 package (10 ounces) frozen mustard greens or frozen cut leaf spinach

1. Combine shrimp, cabbage, celery and green onions in large bowl. Whisk ketchup, horseradish, vinegar, oil, mustard, garlic and salt in small bowl until well blended. Pour over shrimp mixture; toss to coat. Cover and refrigerate at least 15 minutes or up to 2 days.

2. Cook mustard greens according to package directions. Cool, drain and squeeze excess water from greens. Divide greens among serving plates or bowls, top with shrimp salad.

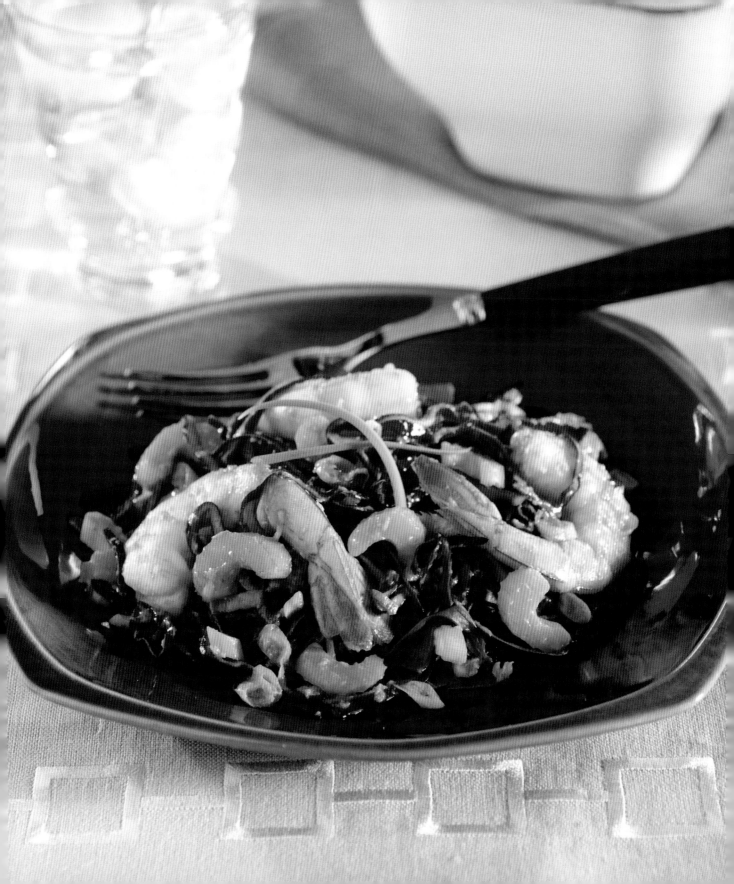

Pan-Cooked
Bok Choy Salmon

makes 2 servings

PER SERVING

410 **calories**
30g **total fat**
8g **carbs**
5g **net carbs**
3g **dietary fiber**
28g **protein**

1   **pound bok choy or napa cabbage, chopped**

1   **cup broccoli slaw mix**

2   **tablespoons olive oil, divided**

2   **salmon fillets (4 to 6 ounces each)**

¼   **teaspoon salt**

¼   **teaspoon black pepper**

1   **teaspoon sesame seeds**

1. Combine bok choy and broccoli slaw mix in colander; rinse and drain well.

2. Heat 1 tablespoon oil in large skillet over medium heat. Sprinkle salmon with ¼ teaspoon salt and ¼ teaspoon pepper. Add salmon to skillet; cook 3 minutes per side. Remove salmon from skillet.

3. Add remaining 1 tablespoon oil and sesame seeds to skillet; stir to toast sesame seeds. Add bok choy mixture; cook and stir 3 to 4 minutes.

4. Return salmon to skillet. Reduce heat to low; cover and cook 4 minutes or until salmon begins to flake when tested with fork. Season with additional salt and pepper, if desired.

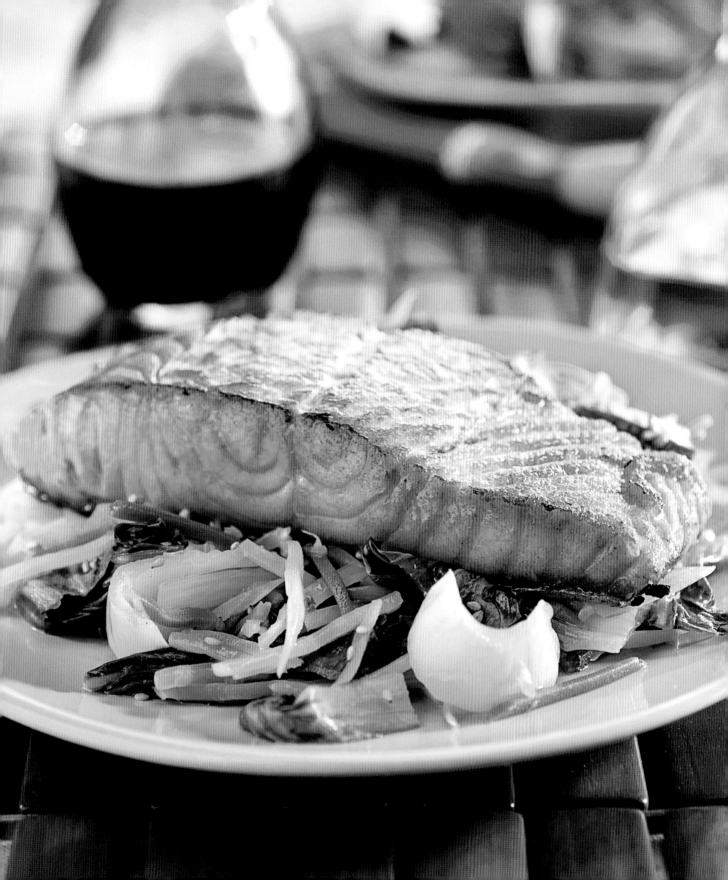

Savoy Shrimp

makes 4 servings

PER SERVING

234 **calories**
9g **total fat**
12g **carbs**
9g **net carbs**
3g **dietary fiber**
25g **protein**

1 **pound large raw shrimp (about 20), peeled and deveined (with tails on)**

½ **teaspoon Chinese five-spice powder**

2 **tablespoons dark sesame oil**

4 **cups sliced savoy or napa cabbage**

1 **cup snow peas, trimmed**

1 **tablespoon soy sauce**

1 **teaspoon red pepper flakes**

½ **teaspoon ground ginger**

Juice of 1 lime

Salt and black pepper

¼ **cup chopped fresh cilantro (optional)**

1. Rinse shrimp; drain well. Toss with Chinese five-spice powder in large bowl.

2. Heat oil in large nonstick skillet over medium heat. Add cabbage, snow peas, soy sauce, red pepper flakes and ground ginger. Cook and stir until cabbage is tender.

3. Add shrimp and lime juice; stir. Cover skillet and reduce heat to low. Cook 3 minutes or until shrimp are pink and opaque. Season with salt and pepper. Garnish with cilantro.

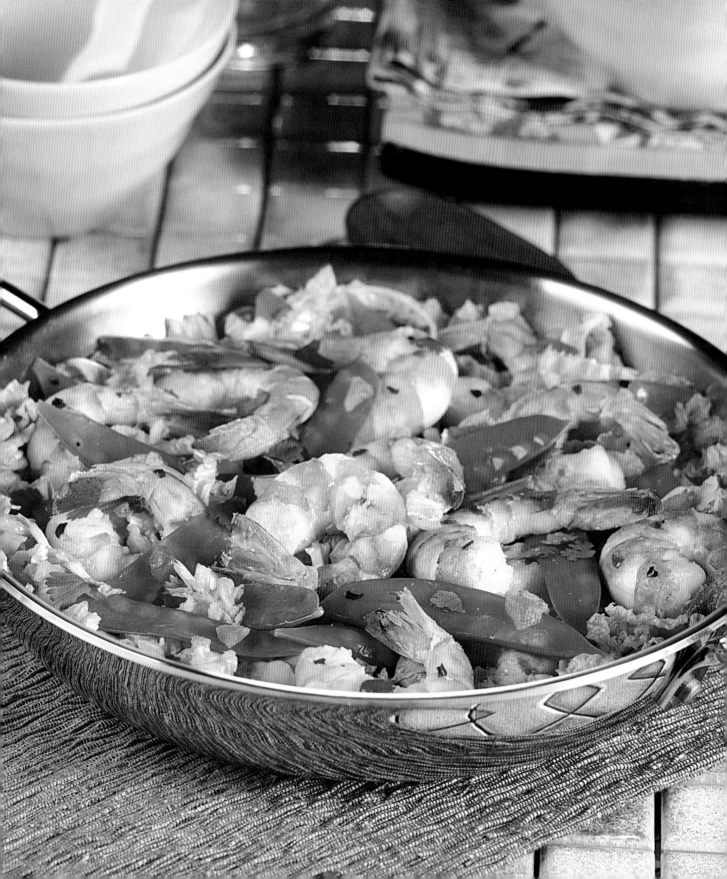

Salmon with Dill-Mustard Sauce

makes 4 servings

PER SERVING

220 calories
12g **total fat**
3g **carbs**
2g **net carbs**
1g **dietary fiber**
23g **protein**

2 tablespoons fresh lemon juice

2 tablespoons fresh lime juice

4 salmon fillets (4 ounces each)

¼ cup mayonnaise

1 tablespoon Dijon mustard

1 tablespoon chopped fresh dill

1. Combine lemon juice and lime juice in glass baking dish. Rinse salmon; pat dry. Place salmon in baking dish; turn to coat evenly. Marinate 10 minutes, turning once.

2. Stir mayonnaise, mustard and dill in small bowl until well blended.

3. Preheat broiler. Spray rack of broiler pan with nonstick cooking spray. Remove salmon from marinade; pat dry. Place on rack.

4. Broil 4 inches from heat source 3 to 4 minutes per side or until salmon begins to flake when tested with fork.

5. Place salmon on serving plates; top with sauce.

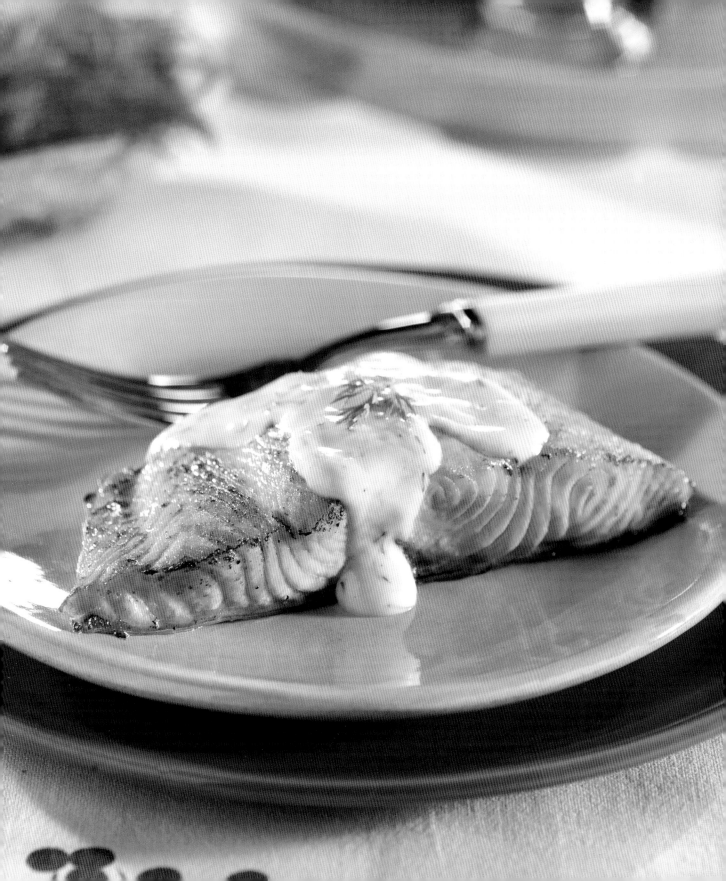

Shrimp and Tomato Stir-Fry

makes 4 servings

20 kalamata olives, pitted and coarsely chopped

1 cup cherry tomatoes, halved

¼ cup chopped fresh basil

¼ teaspoon plus ⅛ teaspoon salt, divided

¼ teaspoon black pepper

1 pound peeled medium raw shrimp

1 clove garlic, minced

⅛ teaspoon red pepper flakes

1 medium zucchini, quartered lengthwise, then cut crosswise into 2-inch pieces

1 medium onion, cut into 8 wedges

1. Combine olives, tomatoes, basil, ⅛ teaspoon salt and pepper in medium bowl; toss gently to blend.

2. Spray large nonstick skillet with nonstick cooking spray; heat over medium heat. Add shrimp, garlic and red pepper flakes; cook and stir 3 minutes or until shrimp are opaque. Transfer to bowl.

3. Spray same skillet with cooking spray; heat over medium-high heat; Add zucchini, onion and remaining ¼ teaspoon salt; cook and stir 5 minutes or until edges of vegetables begin to brown.

4. Add tomato mixture and shrimp to skillet; cook and stir 1 minute or until heated through.

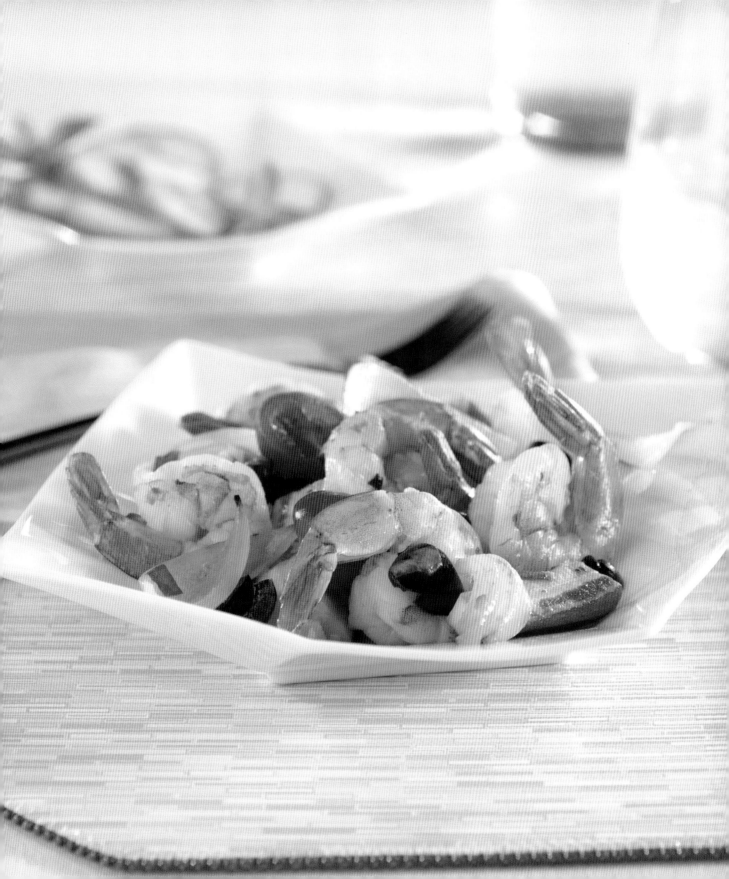

Mustard-Grilled Red Snapper

makes 4 servings

½ cup Dijon mustard

1 tablespoon red wine vinegar

¼ teaspoon ground red pepper

4 red snapper fillets (about
6 ounces each)

1. Spray grid with nonstick cooking spray. Prepare grill for direct cooking.

2. Combine mustard, vinegar and red pepper in small bowl; mix well. Coat fish thoroughly with mustard mixture.

3. Grill fish, covered, over medium-high heat 8 minutes or until fish begins to flake easily when tested with fork, turning halfway through grilling time.

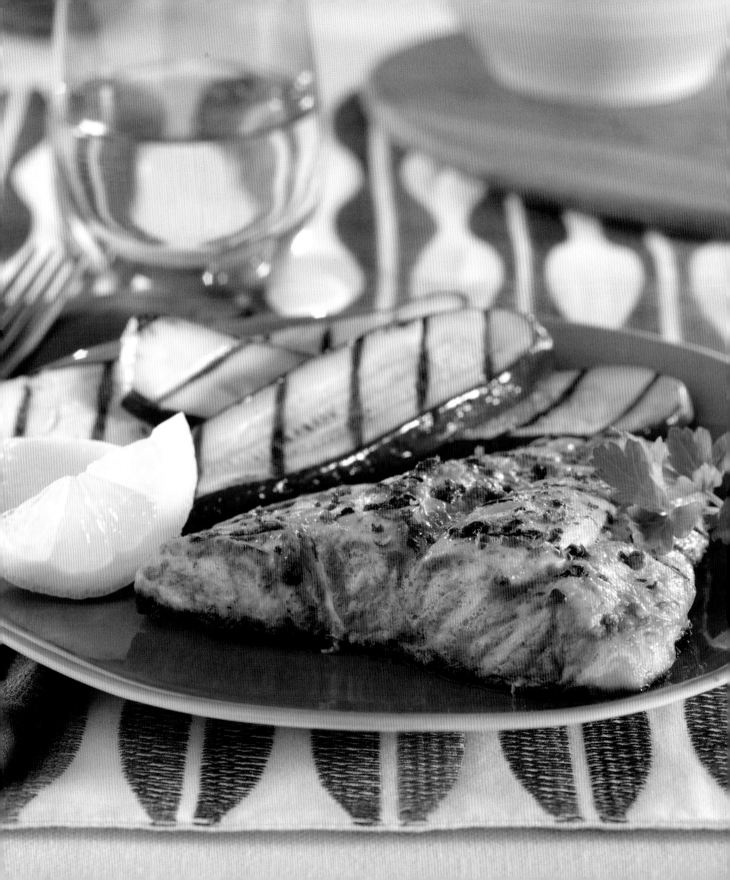

Chipotle Shrimp with Squash Ribbons

makes 4 servings

PER SERVING

139 calories
3g **total fat**
13g **carbs**
10g **net carbs**
3g **dietary fiber**
14g **protein**

2 cloves garlic

1 canned chipotle pepper in adobo sauce, plus 1 teaspoon sauce

2 tablespoons water

2 medium zucchini

2 medium yellow squash

1 teaspoon olive oil

1 small onion, diced

1 medium red bell pepper, cut into strips

8 ounces raw medium shrimp, peeled and deveined

Lime wedges (optional)

1. Place garlic cloves, chipotle pepper, adobo sauce and water in food processor; purée until smooth.

2. Using a vegetable peeler, shave squash into ribbons (discard the seedy middle). Set aside.

3. Heat oil in large skillet over high heat. Add onion and bell pepper; cook and stir 1 minute. Add shrimp and chipotle mixture; cook 2 minutes. Add squash; cook and stir constantly 1 to 2 minutes or until shrimp are no longer pink and squash is heated through and slightly wilted. Serve with lime wedges, if desired.

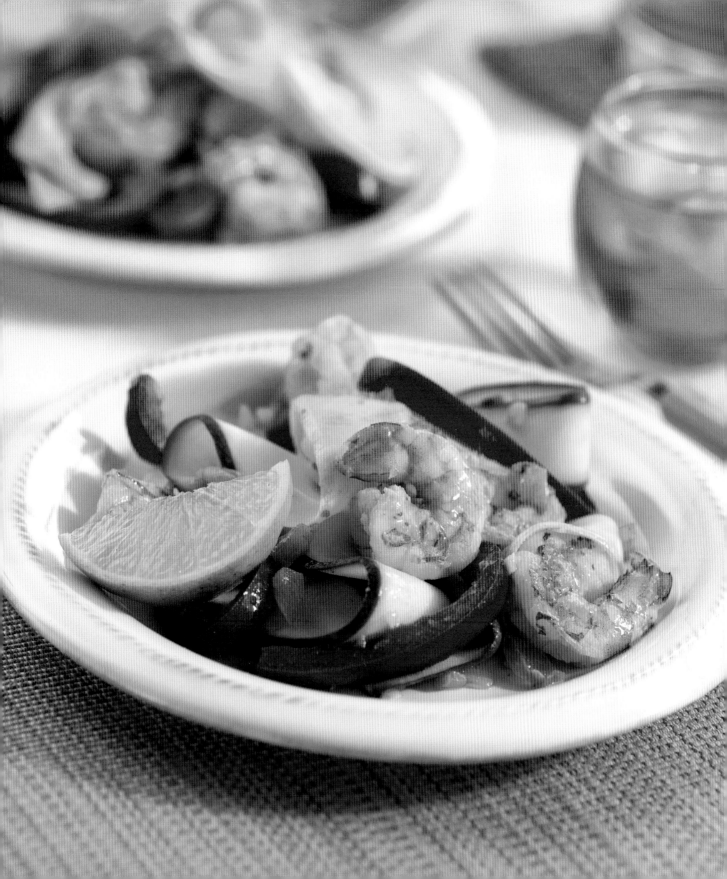

Hazelnut-Coated Salmon Steaks

makes 4 servings

PER SERVING

350 calories
23g **total fat**
2g **carbs**
1g **net carbs**
1g **dietary fiber**
30g **protein**

¼ cup hazelnuts

4 salmon steaks (about 5 ounces each)

1 tablespoon unsweetened applesauce

1 tablespoon Dijon mustard

¼ teaspoon salt

¼ teaspoon dried thyme

⅛ teaspoon black pepper

1. Preheat oven to 375°F. Spread hazelnuts on ungreased baking sheet; bake 8 minutes or until lightly browned. Immediately transfer nuts to clean, dry dish towel. Fold towel over nuts; rub vigorously to remove as much of skins as possible. Finely chop hazelnuts in food processor or with knife.

2. *Increase oven temperature to 450°F.* Place salmon in single layer in baking dish. Combine applesauce, mustard, salt, thyme and pepper in small bowl; brush over salmon. Top with hazelnuts, pressing to adhere.

3. Bake 14 to 16 minutes or until salmon begins to flake when tested with fork.

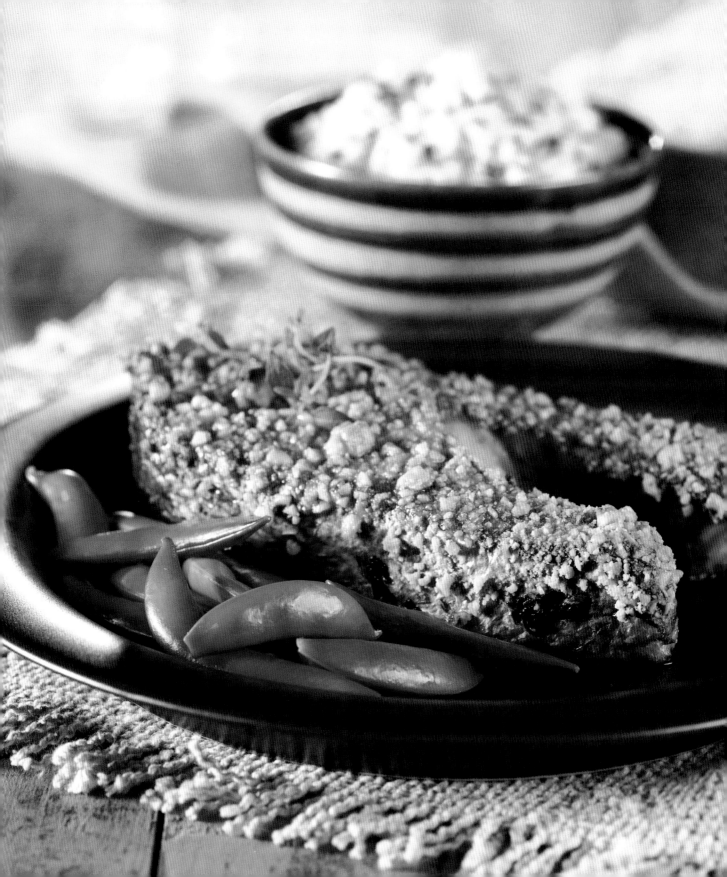

Tuna Teriyaki

makes 4 servings

4 fresh tuna steaks* (about 1½ pounds total)

¼ cup soy sauce

2 tablespoons sake

½ teaspoon minced fresh ginger

¼ teaspoon minced garlic

1½ tablespoons grapeseed oil

2 small limes, cut into halves

Pickled ginger (optional)

Salmon, halibut or swordfish can be substituted for the tuna.

1. Place tuna in shallow dish. Whisk soy sauce, sake, ginger and garlic in small bowl until smooth. Pour over tuna. Cover and marinate in refrigerator 40 minutes, turning frequently.

2. Drain tuna, reserving marinade. Heat oil in large nonstick skillet over medium heat. Add tuna; cook 2 to 3 minutes or until light brown. Turn over; cook 2 to 3 minutes or just until opaque.

3. Reduce heat to medium-low. Pour reserved marinade over tuna. Add limes, cut side down, to skillet. Cook 1 to 1½ minutes or until coated and sauce is bubbly, carefully turning tuna once. Serve with limes and pickled ginger, if desired.

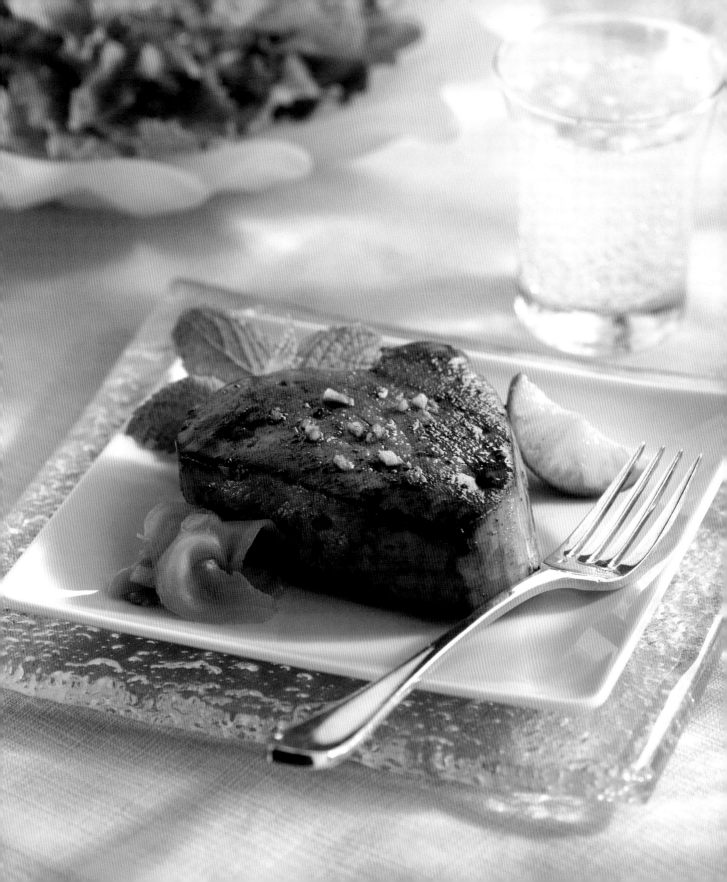

Grilled Salmon Fillets, Asparagus and Onions

makes 6 servings

¼ cup plus 1 tablespoon olive oil, divided

Grated peel and juice of 1 lemon

2 tablespoons Dijon mustard

1 clove garlic, minced

Salt and black pepper

6 salmon fillets (6 to 8 ounces each)

½ teaspoon paprika

1 bunch (about 1 pound) fresh asparagus spears, ends trimmed

1 large red or sweet onion, cut into ¼-inch slices

1. Prepare grill for direct grilling. Whisk ¼ cup oil, lemon peel and juice, mustard and garlic in medium bowl. Season with salt and pepper.

2. Place salmon on large plate or sheet pan. Sprinkle with paprika and brush evenly with Dijon mixture; let stand at room temperature 15 minutes.

3. Brush asparagus and onion slices with remaining 1 tablespoon oil; season with salt and pepper.

4. Place salmon, skin side down, in center of grid. Place asparagus and onion slices around salmon. Grill, covered, 5 minutes. Turn salmon and vegetables. Grill 5 to 6 minutes more or until salmon flakes when tested with fork and vegetables are crisp-tender. Separate onion slices into rings.

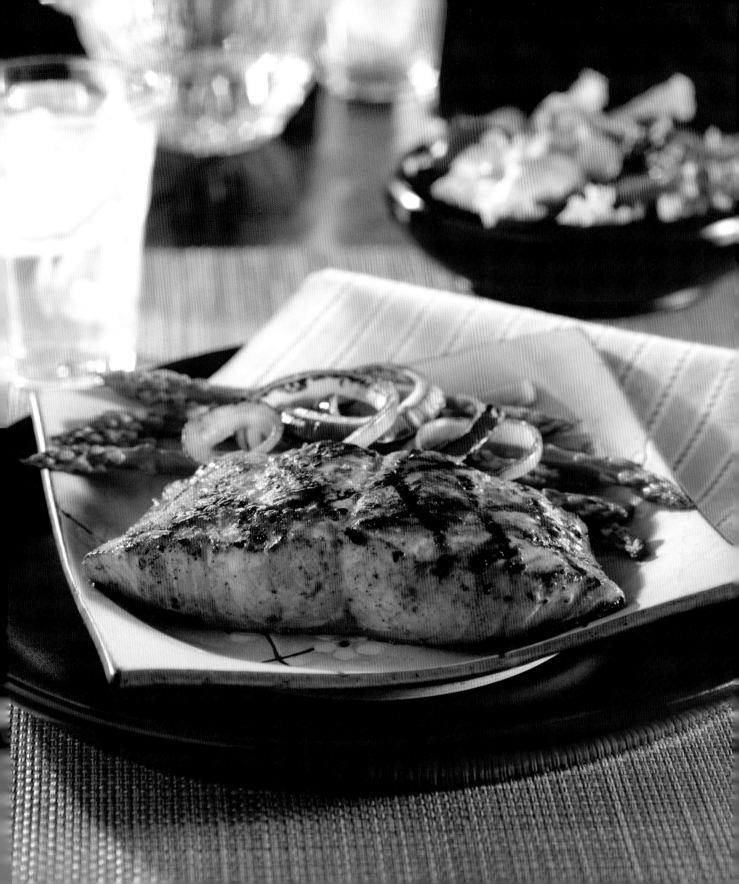

Shrimp Pâté

makes 1½ cups spread (2 tablespoons per serving)

8 ounces cooked peeled shrimp

¼ cup (½ stick) unsalted butter, cut into chunks

2 teaspoons dry vermouth or chicken broth

1 teaspoon lemon juice

1 teaspoon Dijon mustard

¼ teaspoon salt

¼ teaspoon ground mace

⅛ teaspoon ground red pepper

⅛ teaspoon black pepper

½ cup chopped shelled pistachios

2 large heads Belgian endive

1. Combine shrimp, butter, vermouth, lemon juice, mustard, salt, mace, red pepper and black pepper in blender or food processor. Process until smooth. Shape mixture into 8-inch log on waxed paper. (If mixture is too soft to handle refrigerate 1 hour.)

2. Spread pistachios on sheet of waxed paper. Roll pâté log in nuts to coat. Cover and refrigerate 1 to 3 hours.

3. Separate endive into individual leaves. Place pâté on serving plate; serve with endive leaves.

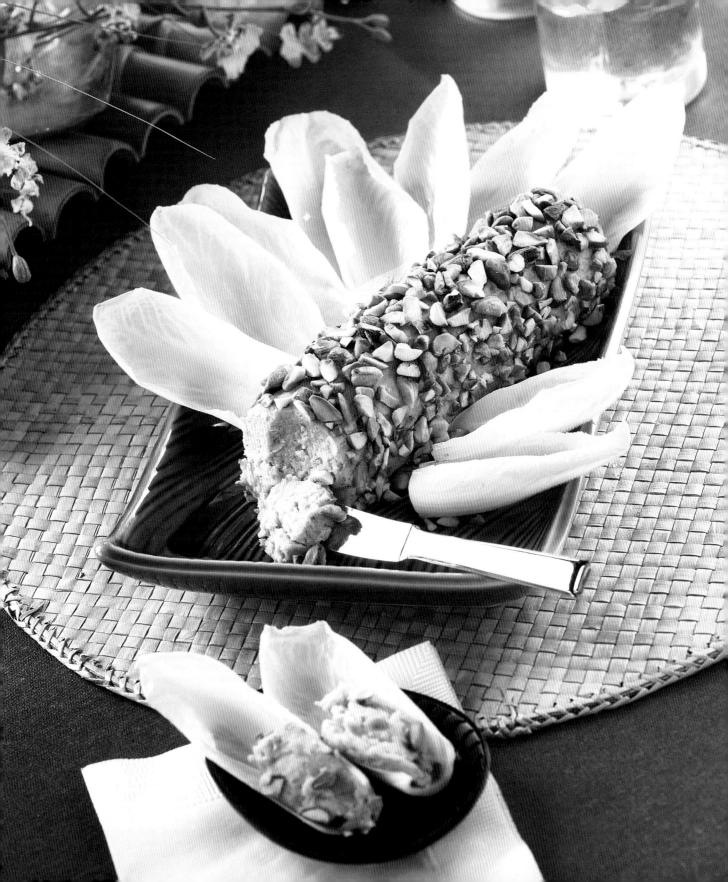

Broiled Trout with Pine Nut Butter

makes 4 servings

4 whole trout (each about 8 ounces), cleaned

¼ cup olive oil

¼ cup dry white wine

2 tablespoons minced fresh chives

2 tablespoons chopped fresh parsley

½ teaspoon salt

⅛ teaspoon black pepper

¼ cup (½ stick) butter, softened

¼ cup pine nuts, finely chopped

1. Place trout in large resealable food storage bag. Whisk oil, wine, chives, parsley, salt and pepper in small bowl. Pour over fish; seal bag. Marinate in refrigerator 30 minutes or up to 2 hours, turning occasionally.

2. Combine butter and pine nuts in small bowl; stir until well blended. Cover; let stand at room temperature until ready to use.

3. Preheat broiler; spray broiling pan with nonstick cooking spray. Remove fish from marinade; reserve marinade. Place fish on broiler pan. Broil 4 to 6 inches from heat 4 minutes; turn fish over. Brush with marinade; broil 4 to 6 minutes or until fish turns opaque and just begins to flake when tested with fork. Transfer fish to serving platter. Top with butter mixture.

Note: If you prefer to grill trout, place fish in a hinged wire basket and grill, uncovered, 4 to 6 inches over medium heat.

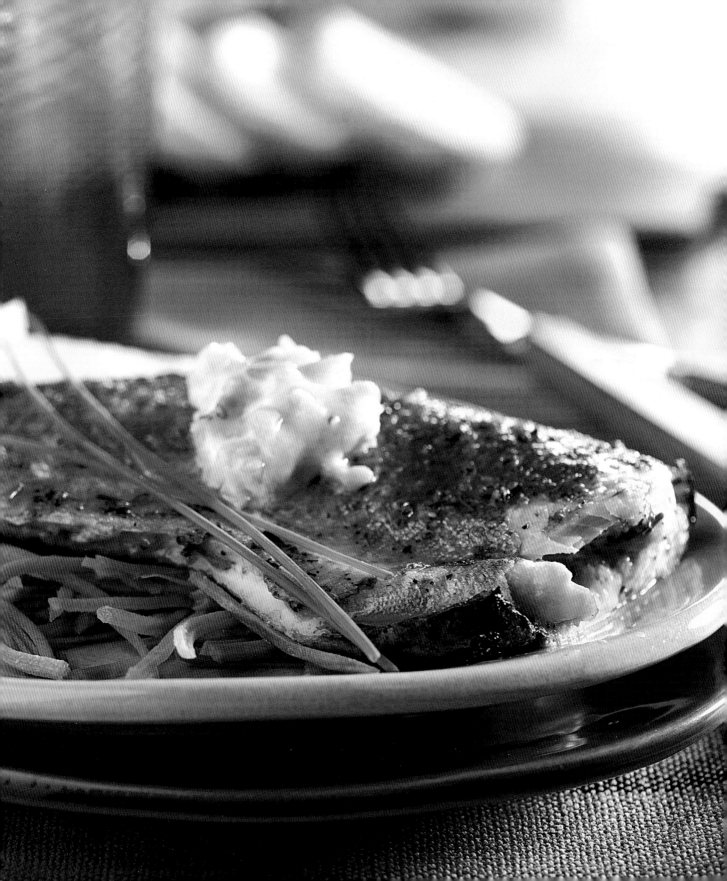

Shrimp Scampi

makes 8 servings

PER SERVING

150 **calories**
10g **total fat**
3g **carbs**
3g **net carbs**
0g **dietary fiber**
12g **protein**

¼ cup (½ stick) plus 2 tablespoons butter

6 to 8 cloves garlic, minced

1½ pounds large raw shrimp (about 16), peeled and deveined

6 green onions, thinly sliced

¼ cup dry white wine or chicken broth

Juice of 1 lemon (about 2 tablespoons)

¼ cup chopped fresh parsley

Salt and black pepper

Lemon slices (optional)

1. Clarify butter by melting it in small saucepan over low heat. *Do not stir.* Skim off white foam that forms on top. Strain clarified butter through cheesecloth into glass measuring cup to yield ⅓ cup. Discard cheesecloth and milky residue at bottom of pan.

2. Heat clarified butter in large skillet over medium heat. Add garlic; cook and stir 1 to 2 minutes or until softened but not browned.

3. Add shrimp, green onions, wine and lemon juice; cook and stir 3 to 4 minutes or until shrimp are pink and opaque. *Do not overcook.*

4. Stir in parsley and season with salt and pepper. Garnish with lemon slices.

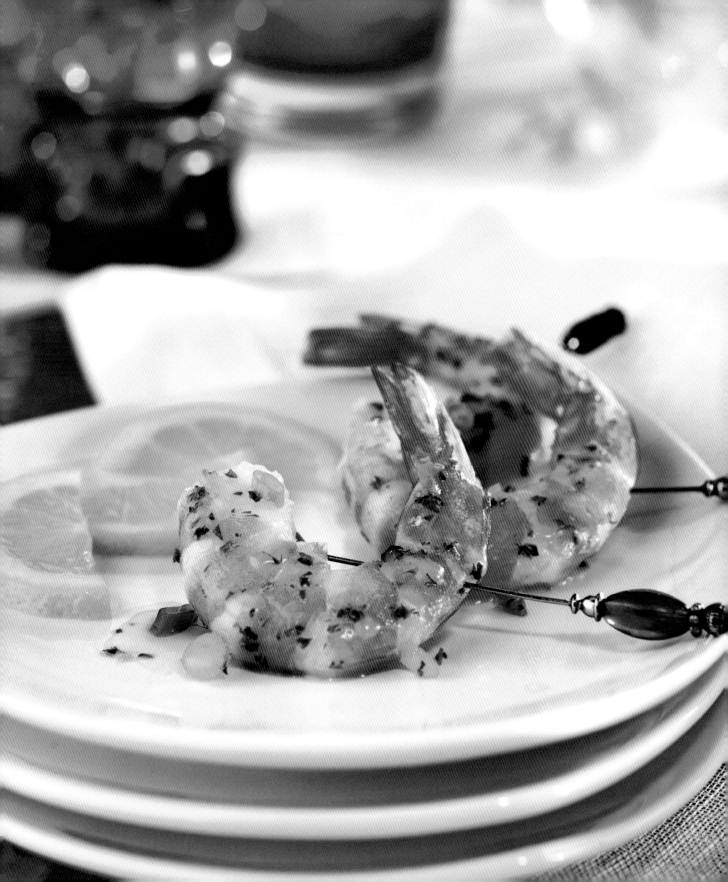

Grilled Chinese Salmon

makes 4 servings

3 tablespoons soy sauce

2 tablespoons dry sherry

2 cloves garlic, minced

4 salmon fillet pieces or steaks
   (about 1 pound)

2 tablespoons finely chopped
   fresh cilantro

1. Combine soy sauce, sherry and garlic in shallow dish. Add salmon; turn to coat. Cover and marinate in refrigerator at least 30 minutes or up to 2 hours.

2. Oil grid. Prepare grill for direct cooking.

3. Remove salmon from dish, reserving marinade. Arrange fillets, skin side down, on oiled grid over high heat or on oiled rack of broiler pan. Grill or broil 10 minutes or until center is opaque, basting with reserved marinade after 5 minutes of cooking. Discard any remaining marinade. Sprinkle with cilantro.

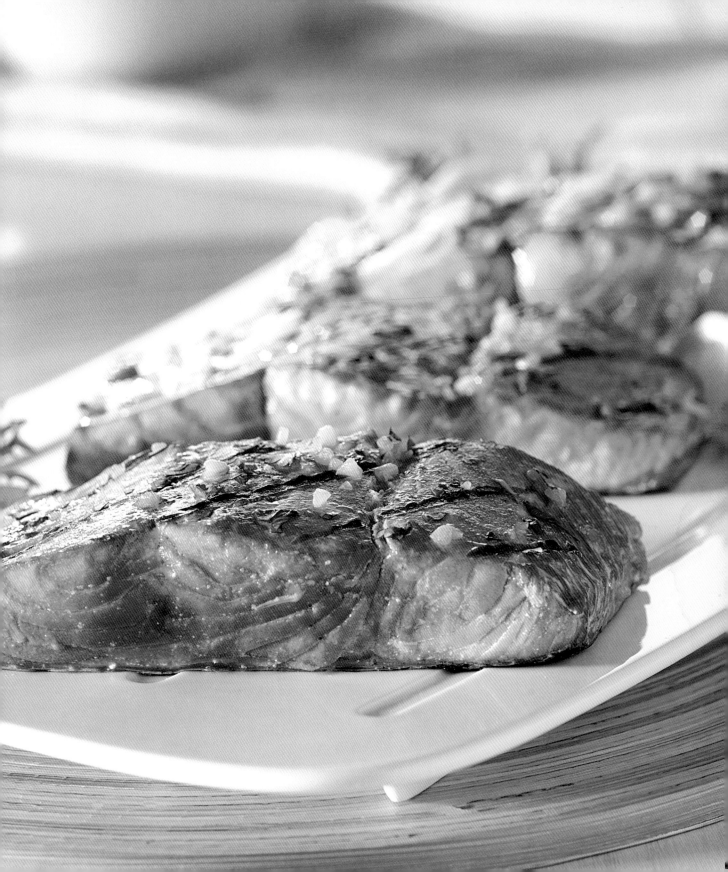

Grilled Lobster, Shrimp and Calamari Ceviche

makes 6 servings

¾ cup orange juice

⅓ cup fresh lime juice

2 jalapeño peppers, seeded and minced

2 tablespoons chopped fresh cilantro, chives or green onion tops

2 tablespoons tequila

1 teaspoon ground cumin

1 teaspoon olive oil

10 squid, cleaned and cut into rings and tentacles

8 ounces medium raw shrimp, peeled and deveined

2 lobster tails (8 ounces each), meat removed and shells discarded

1. For marinade, combine orange juice, lime juice, jalapeños, cilantro and tequila in medium bowl.

2. Measure ¼ cup marinade into small bowl; stir in cumin and oil. Reserve. Refrigerate remaining marinade.

3. Prepare grill for direct cooking.

4. Bring 1 quart water to a boil in large saucepan over high heat. Add squid; cook 30 seconds or until opaque. Drain and rinse under cold water. Add squid to refrigerated marinade.

5. Thread shrimp onto metal skewers. Brush shrimp and lobster with reserved ¼ cup marinade.

6. Place shrimp on grid. Grill shrimp, uncovered, over medium-high heat 2 to 3 minutes per side or until pink and opaque. Remove shrimp from skewers; add to squid. Place lobster on grid. Grill 5 minutes per side or until meat turns opaque and is cooked through. Cut lobster meat into ¼-inch-thick slices; add to squid and shrimp mixture.

7. Refrigerate at least 2 hours or overnight.

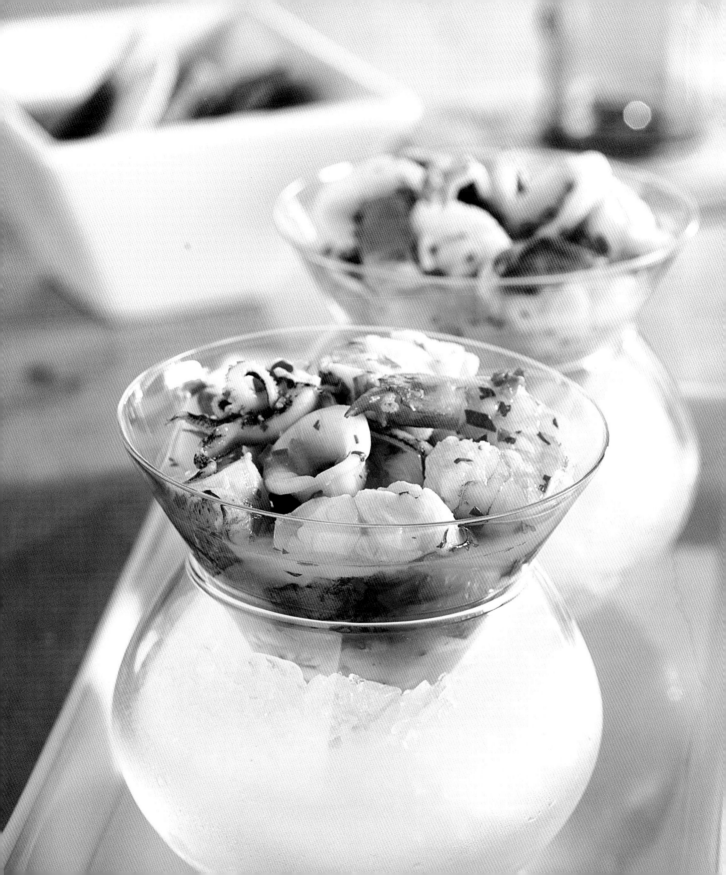

Catfish with Bacon and Horseradish

makes 6 servings

PER SERVING

380 calories
30g **total fat**
4g **carbs**
4g **net carbs**
0g **dietary fiber**
22g **protein**

6 farm-raised catfish fillets (4 to 5 ounces each)

2 tablespoons butter

¼ cup chopped onion

1 package (8 ounces) cream cheese, softened

¼ cup dry white wine or vegetable broth

2 tablespoons prepared horseradish

1 tablespoon Dijon mustard

½ teaspoon salt

⅛ teaspoon black pepper

4 slices bacon, crisp-cooked and crumbled

1. Preheat oven to 350°F. Grease large baking dish. Arrange fillets in single layer in prepared dish.

2. Melt butter in small skillet over medium-high heat. Add onion; cook and stir 5 minutes or until softened. Combine cream cheese, wine, horseradish, mustard, salt and pepper in medium bowl; stir in onion. Pour over fish and top with crumbled bacon.

3. Bake 30 minutes or until fish begins to flake when tested with fork.

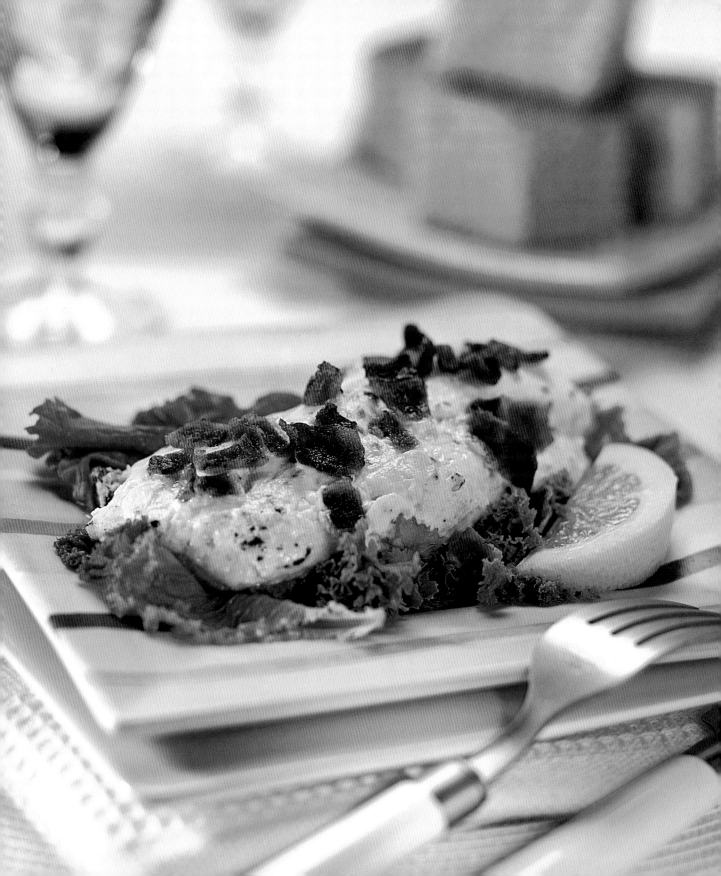

Salmon Burgers with Tarragon Aïoli

makes 4 servings

PER SERVING

190 **calories**
14g **total fat**
6g **carbs**
4g **net carbs**
2g **dietary fiber**
11g **protein**

Tarragon Aïoli

- ⅓ cup sour cream
- 1½ tablespoons mayonnaise
- 1 tablespoon milk
- ½ teaspoon dried tarragon
- ¼ teaspoon salt
- ⅛ teaspoon black pepper

Burgers

- 1 can (6 ounces) pink salmon, drained
- ¼ cup almond flour
- ⅓ cup chopped green onions
- ¼ cup chopped fresh cilantro
- 2 egg whites
- 2 tablespoons lime juice
- ¼ teaspoon salt
- ⅛ teaspoon ground red pepper

1. For aïoli, combine sour cream, mayonnaise, cream, tarragon, ¼ teaspoon salt and black pepper in medium bowl. Refrigerate until ready to use.

2. For burgers, combine salmon, almond flour, green onions, cilantro, egg whites, lime juice and red pepper in large bowl; mix well.

3. Coat large nonstick skillet with nonstick cooking spray; heat over medium heat. Spoon equal amounts of salmon mixture into 4 mounds in skillet. Using a flat spatula, flatten each mound. Cook 3 minutes on each side or until golden. Serve with sauce.

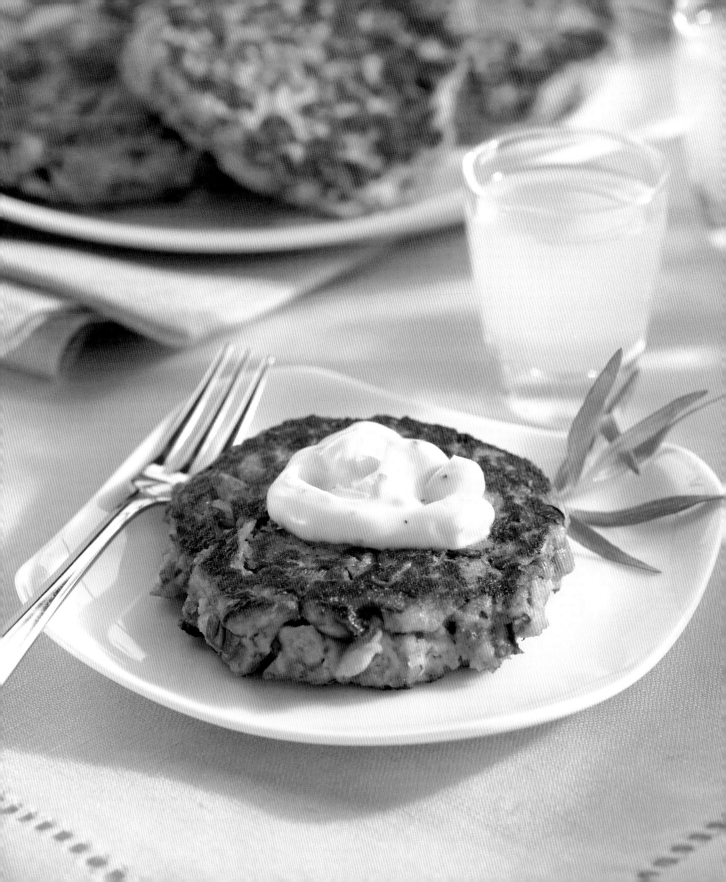

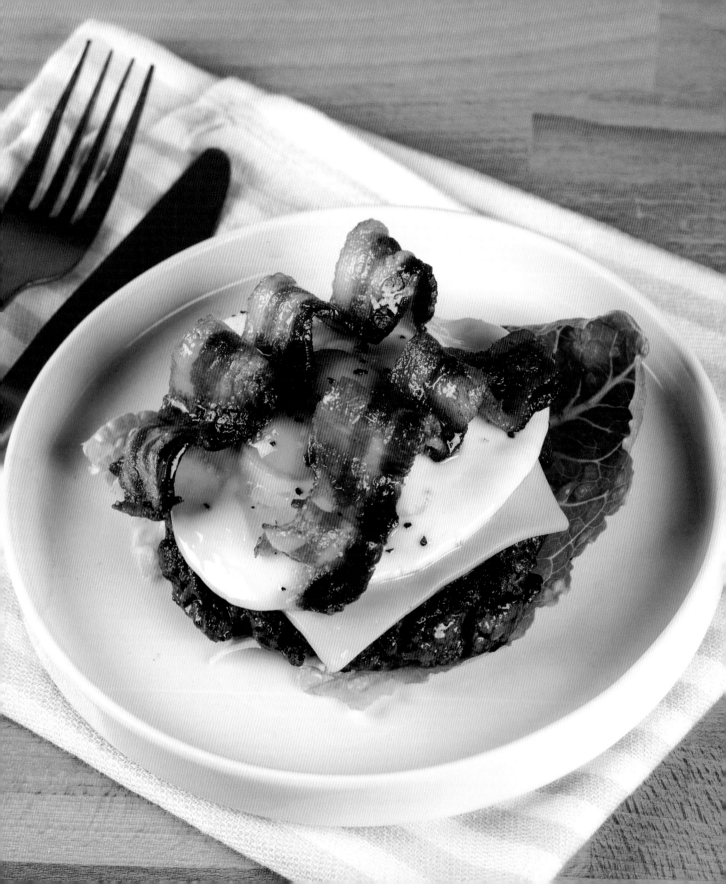

comfort food

Bacon Smashburger

makes 4 servings

4 slices bacon, cut in half
1 pound ground chuck
   Salt and black pepper
4 slices sharp Cheddar cheese
4 eggs (optional)

1. Cook bacon in large skillet over medium-high heat until crisp. Remove from skillet; drain on paper towels. Drain all but 1 tablespoon drippings from skillet.

2. Divide beef into 4 portions and shape lightly into loose balls. Place in same skillet over medium-high heat. Smash with spatula to flatten into thin patties; sprinkle with salt and pepper. Cook 2 to 3 minutes or until edges and bottoms are browned. Flip burgers and top with cheese. Cook 2 to 3 minutes for medium rare or to desired degree of doneness. Transfer to plates.

3. If desired, crack eggs into hot skillet. Cook over medium heat about 3 minutes or until whites are opaque and yolks are desired degree of doneness, flipping once, if desired, for overeasy. Place on burgers; top with bacon.

Spinach Artichoke Gratin

makes 6 servings

PER SERVING

125 calories
1g total fat
13g carbs
8g net carbs
5g dietary fiber
15g protein

2 cups (16 ounces) cottage cheese

2 eggs, beaten

4½ tablespoons grated Parmesan cheese, divided

1 tablespoon lemon juice

⅛ teaspoon black pepper

⅛ teaspoon ground nutmeg

2 packages (10 ounces each) frozen chopped spinach, thawed

⅓ cup thinly sliced green onions

1 package (10 ounces) frozen artichoke hearts, thawed and halved

1. Preheat oven to 375°F. Spray 1½-quart baking dish with nonstick cooking spray.

2. Combine cottage cheese, eggs, 3 tablespoons Parmesan cheese, lemon juice, pepper and nutmeg in food processor or blender; process until smooth.

3. Squeeze moisture from spinach. Combine spinach, cottage cheese mixture and green onions in large bowl; mix well. Spread half of mixture in prepared baking dish.

4. Pat artichokes dry with paper towels; place in single layer over spinach mixture. Sprinkle with remaining 1½ tablespoons Parmesan cheese. Cover with remaining spinach mixture.

5. Cover and bake 25 minutes.

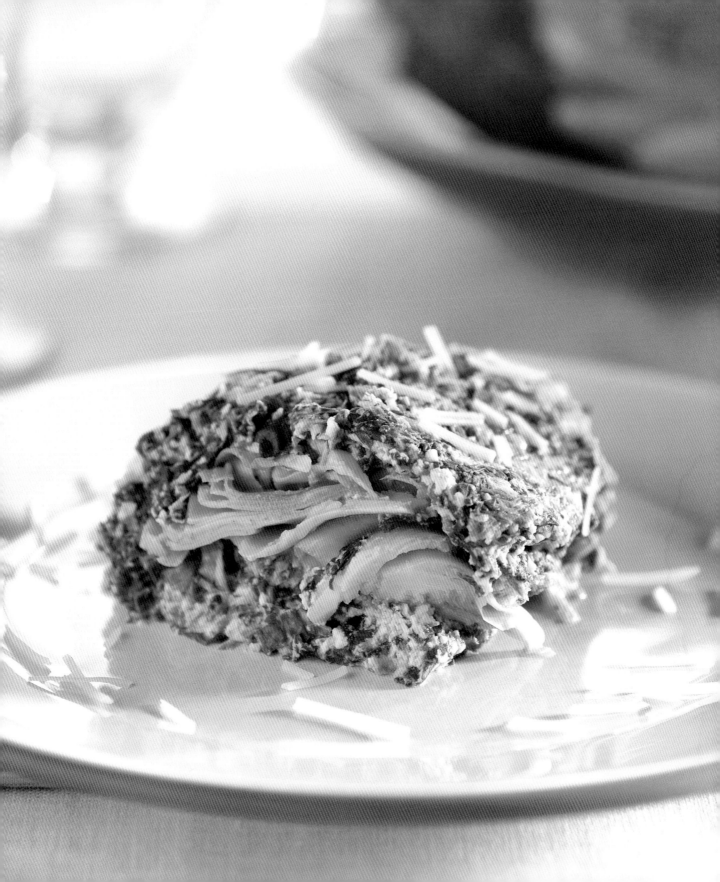

Noodle-Free Lasagna

makes 8 servings

PER SERVING

443 calories
34g **total fat**
16g **carbs**
11g **net carbs**
5g **dietary fiber**
24g **protein**

1 medium eggplant

2 medium zucchini

2 medium yellow squash

1¼ pounds lean sweet Italian turkey sausage, casings removed

2 medium bell peppers, diced

2 cups mushrooms, thinly sliced

1 can (about 14 ounces) diced tomatoes

1 cup tomato sauce

½ cup chopped fresh basil

1 teaspoon dried oregano

½ teaspoon salt

¼ teaspoon black pepper

1 container (15 ounces) whole-milk ricotta cheese

2 cups (8 ounces) shredded mozzarella cheese

¼ cup grated Parmesan cheese

1. Preheat oven to 375°F. Cut eggplant, zucchini and yellow squash lengthwise into ⅛-inch slices. Place on baking sheet. Bake 10 minutes. Set aside to cool.

2. Heat large nonstick skillet over medium-high heat. Add sausage; cook 8 to 10 minutes or until cooked through, stirring to break up meat. Drain fat. Transfer to plate.

3. Add bell peppers and mushrooms to skillet; cook and stir 3 to 4 minutes or until vegetables are tender. Return sausage to skillet. Add tomatoes, tomato sauce, basil, oregano, salt and black pepper; cook and stir 1 to 2 minutes or until heated through.

4. Spray 13×9-inch baking pan with nonstick cooking spray. Layer one third of eggplant, zucchini and yellow squash in prepared pan. Spread half of ricotta cheese over vegetables. Top with one third of tomato sauce mixture. Sprinkle evenly with half of mozzarella cheese. Repeat layers once, ending with final layer of vegetables and tomato sauce mixture. Sprinkle with Parmesan cheese; cover with foil.

5. Bake 45 minutes. Remove foil; bake 10 to 15 minutes or until vegetables are tender. Let stand 10 minutes before cutting.

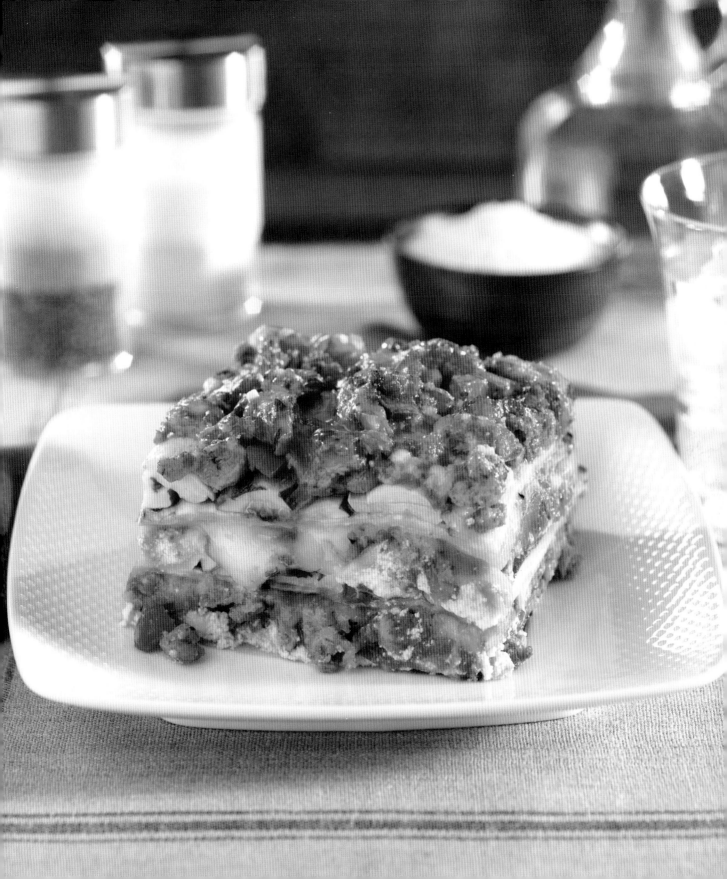

Bacon-Tomato Grilled Cheese

makes 4 servings

PER SERVING

530 calories
45g total fat
10g carbs
7g net carbs
3g dietary fiber
27g protein

8 slices bacon, cut in half

4 slices sharp Cheddar cheese

4 slices Gouda cheese

4 tomato slices, cut in half

½ loaf keto bread (page 194), cut into 8 slices

1 tablespoon butter

1. Cook bacon in large skillet over medium-high heat until crisp. Remove from skillet; drain on paper towels. Drain drippings from skillet; wipe out skillet with paper towels.

2. For each sandwich, layer 1 slice of Cheddar cheese, 1 slice of Gouda cheese, 2 tomato slices and 4 bacon slices between two bread slices.

3. Melt butter in same skillet over medium heat. Add sandwiches; cook 3 to 4 minutes or until bottoms are toasted. Flip sandwiches. Reduce heat to medium-low; cover and cook 3 to 4 minutes or until bottoms are toasted and cheese is melted.

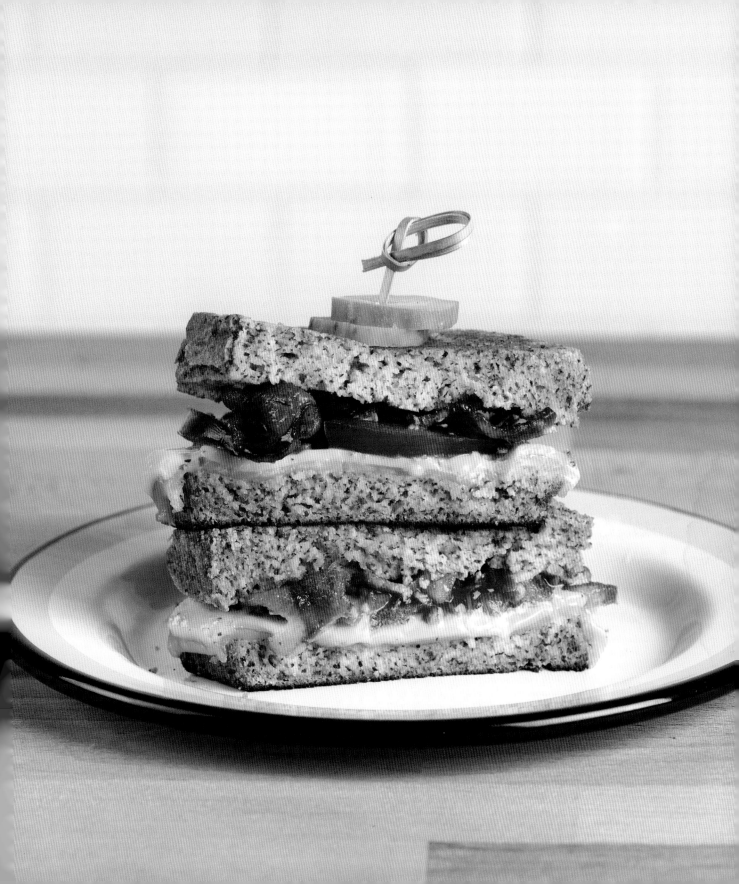

Moussaka

makes 6 servings

PER SERVING

306 **calories**
19g **total fat**
12g **carbs**
9g **net carbs**
3g **dietary fiber**
20g **protein**

1 **eggplant (about 1 pound), cut into ¼-inch slices**

2 **tablespoons olive oil**

1 **pound ground beef**

1 **can (about 14 ounces) stewed tomatoes, drained**

¼ **cup red wine**

2 **tablespoons tomato paste**

¾ **teaspoon salt**

½ **teaspoon dried oregano**

¼ **teaspoon ground cinnamon**

¼ **teaspoon black pepper**

⅛ **teaspoon ground allspice**

4 **ounces cream cheese**

¼ **cup milk**

¼ **cup grated Parmesan cheese**

Additional ground cinnamon (optional)

1. Preheat broiler. Lightly coat 8-inch square baking dish with nonstick cooking spray.

2. Line baking sheet with foil. Arrange eggplant slices on foil, overlapping slightly if necessary. Brush with oil; broil 5 to 6 inches from heat 4 minutes on each side. *Reduce oven temperature to 350°F.*

3. Meanwhile, brown beef in large nonstick skillet over medium-high heat 6 to 8 minutes, stirring to break up meat. Drain fat. Add tomatoes, wine, tomato paste, salt, oregano, ¼ teaspoon cinnamon, pepper and allspice. Bring to a boil, breaking up large pieces of tomato with spoon. Reduce heat to medium-low; cover and simmer 10 minutes.

4. Place cream cheese and milk in small microwavable bowl. Cover and microwave on HIGH 1 minute. Stir until smooth.

5. Arrange half of eggplant slices in prepared baking dish. Spoon half of meat sauce over eggplant; sprinkle with half of Parmesan cheese. Repeat layers. Spoon cream cheese mixture evenly over top. Bake 20 minutes or until top begins to crack slightly. Sprinkle lightly with additional cinnamon, if desired. Let stand 10 minutes before serving.

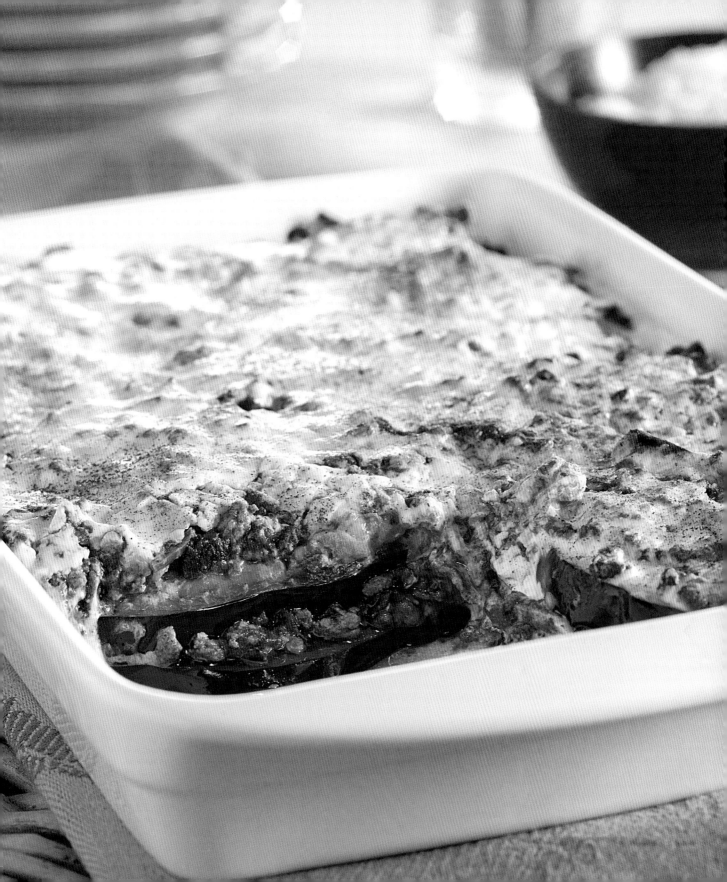

Tuna Melt

makes 4 servings

PER SERVING

980 calories
80g **total fat**
9g **carbs**
6g **net carbs**
3g **dietary fiber**
62g **protein**

¾ cup mayonnaise

2 teaspoons lemon juice

1 teaspoon salt

⅛ teaspoon black pepper

1 can (12 ounces) solid white albacore tuna, drained

1 can (12 ounces) chunk light tuna, drained

1 stalk celery, finely chopped (about ½ cup)

¼ cup minced red onion

½ loaf keto bread (page 194), cut into 8 slices

8 slices Cheddar cheese

2 tablespoons butter

Optional toppings: tomato slices, onion slices, sliced avocado, pickles and/or lettuce leaves

1. Combine mayonnaise, lemon juice, salt and pepper in large bowl. Add tuna, celery and red onion; mix well.

2. Divide tuna among bread slices; top each with cheese. Heat 1 tablespoon butter in large skillet over medium heat until melted. Add half of sandwiches; cover and cook until bread is toasted and cheese is softened. Repeat with remaining butter and sandwiches. Garnish with desired toppings.

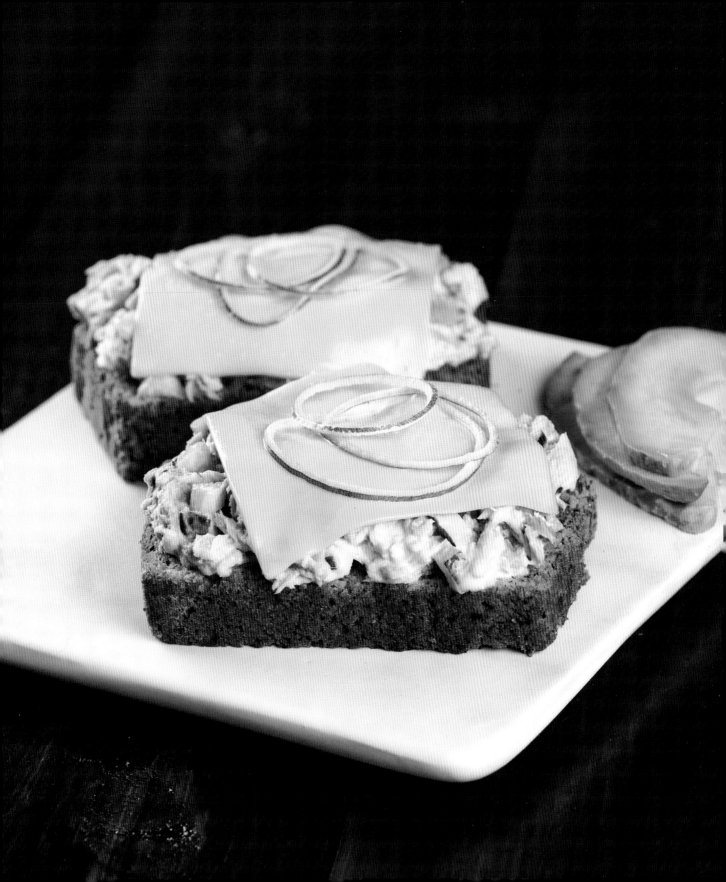

Two-Cheese Sausage Pizza

makes 4 servings

1 pound sweet Italian turkey sausage

1 tablespoon olive oil

2 cups sliced mushrooms

1 small red onion, thinly sliced

1 small green bell pepper, cut into thin strips

¼ teaspoon salt

¼ teaspoon dried oregano

¼ teaspoon black pepper

½ cup pizza sauce

2 tablespoons tomato paste

½ cup shredded Parmesan cheese

1 cup (4 ounces) shredded mozzarella cheese

8 pitted black olives

1. Preheat oven to 400°F. Remove sausage from casings. Pat into 9-inch glass pie plate. Bake 10 minutes or until sausage is firm. Remove from oven and carefully pour off fat. Set aside.

2. Heat oil in large skillet over medium-high heat. Add mushrooms, onion, bell pepper, salt, oregano and black pepper; cook and stir 10 minutes or until vegetables are very tender.

3. Combine pizza sauce and tomato paste in small bowl; stir until well blended. Spread over sausage crust. Spoon half of vegetables over tomato sauce. Sprinkle with Parmesan and mozzarella cheeses. Top with remaining vegetables. Sprinkle with olives. Bake 8 to 10 minutes or until cheese melts.

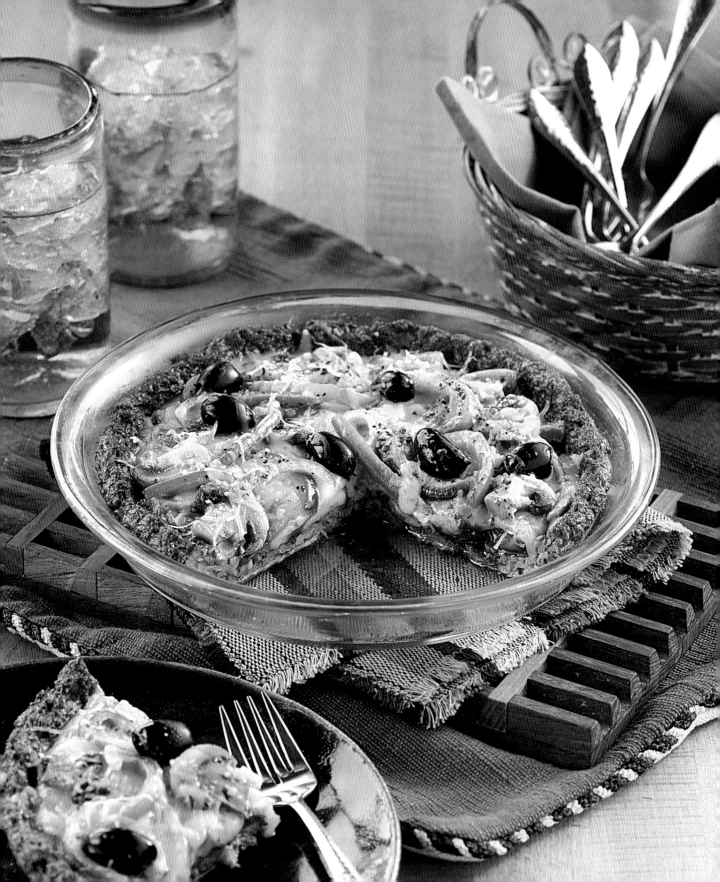

Keto Bread

makes 1 loaf (16 slices)

PER SERVING

156 **calories**
13g **total fat**
4g **carbs**
2g **net carbs**
2g **dietary fiber**
5g **protein**

 7 **tablespoons butter, divided**
 2 **cups almond flour**
3½ **teaspoons baking powder**
 ½ **teaspoon salt**
 6 **eggs, at room temperature, separated***
 ¼ **teaspoon cream of tartar**

Discard 1 egg yolk.

1. Preheat oven to 375°F. Generously grease 8×4-inch loaf pan with 1 tablespoon butter. Melt remaining 6 tablespoons butter; cool slightly.

2. Combine almond flour, baking powder and salt in medium bowl. Add melted butter and 5 egg yolks; stir until blended.

3. Place egg whites and cream of tartar in bowl of stand mixer; attach whip attachment to mixer. Whip egg whites on high speed 1 to 2 minutes or until stiff peaks form.

4. Stir one third of egg whites into almond flour mixture until well blended. Gently fold in remaining egg whites until thoroughly blended. Scrape batter into prepared pan; smooth top.

5. Bake 25 to 30 minutes or until top is light brown and dry and toothpick inserted into center comes out clean. Cool in pan on wire rack 10 minutes. Remove from pan; cool completely.

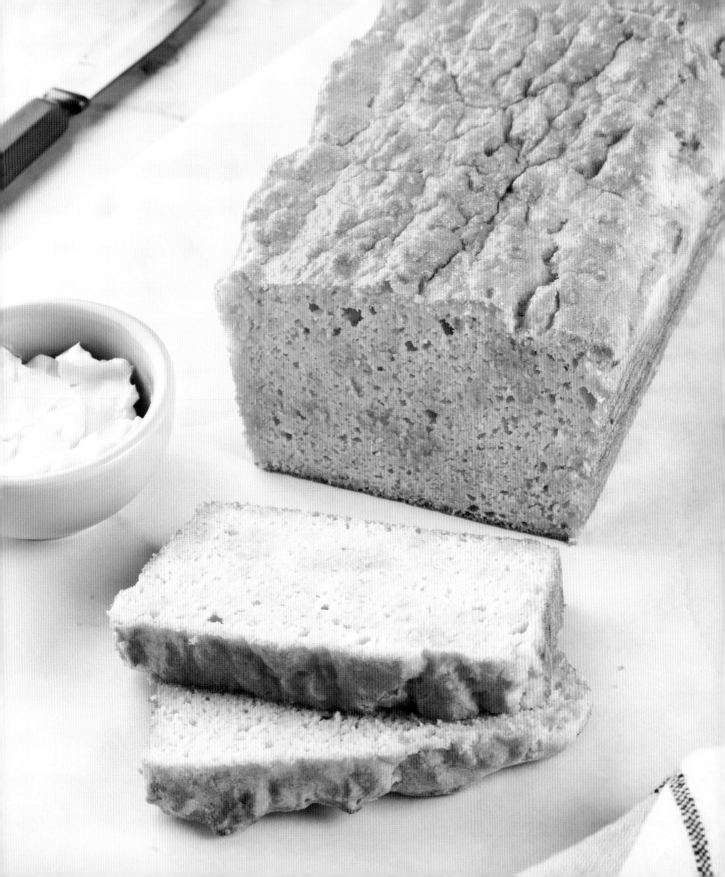

Pesto Turkey Meatballs

makes 4 servings

PER SERVING

390 calories
23g total fat
12g carbs
8g net carbs
4g dietary fiber
37g protein

1 pound ground turkey

⅓ cup prepared pesto

⅓ cup grated Parmesan cheese

¼ cup almond flour

1 egg

2 green onions, finely chopped

½ teaspoon salt, divided

2 tablespoons olive oil

2 cloves garlic, minced

⅛ teaspoon red pepper flakes

1 can (28 ounces) whole tomatoes, crushed with hands or coarsely chopped, juice reserved

1 tablespoon tomato paste

Cooked zucchini noodles (optional)

1. Combine turkey, pesto, cheese, almond flour, egg, green onions and ¼ teaspoon salt in medium bowl; mix well. Shape mixture into 24 balls (about 1¼ inches). Refrigerate meatballs while preparing sauce.

2. Heat oil in large saucepan or Dutch oven over medium heat. Add garlic and red pepper flakes; cook and stir 2 minutes. Add tomatoes with liquid, tomato paste and remaining ¼ teaspoon salt; cook 5 minutes or until sauce begins to simmer, stirring occasionally.

3. Remove about 1 cup sauce from saucepan. Arrange meatballs in single layer in saucepan; pour reserved sauce over meatballs. Reduce heat to medium-low; cover and cook 20 minutes.

4. Uncover; increase heat to medium-high. Cook about 10 minutes or until sauce thickens slightly and meatballs are cooked through. Serve over zucchini noodles, if desired.

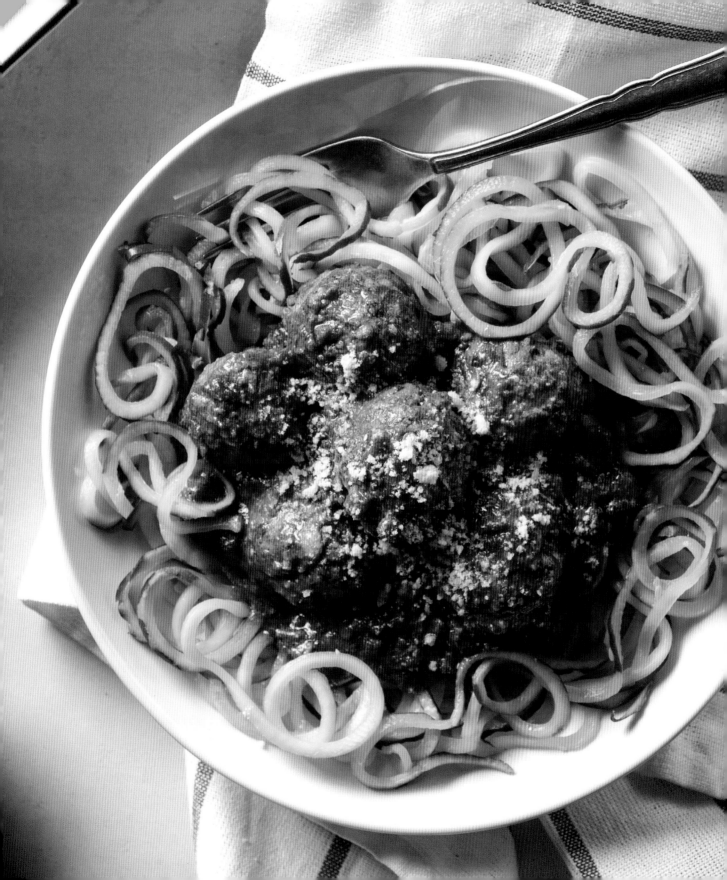

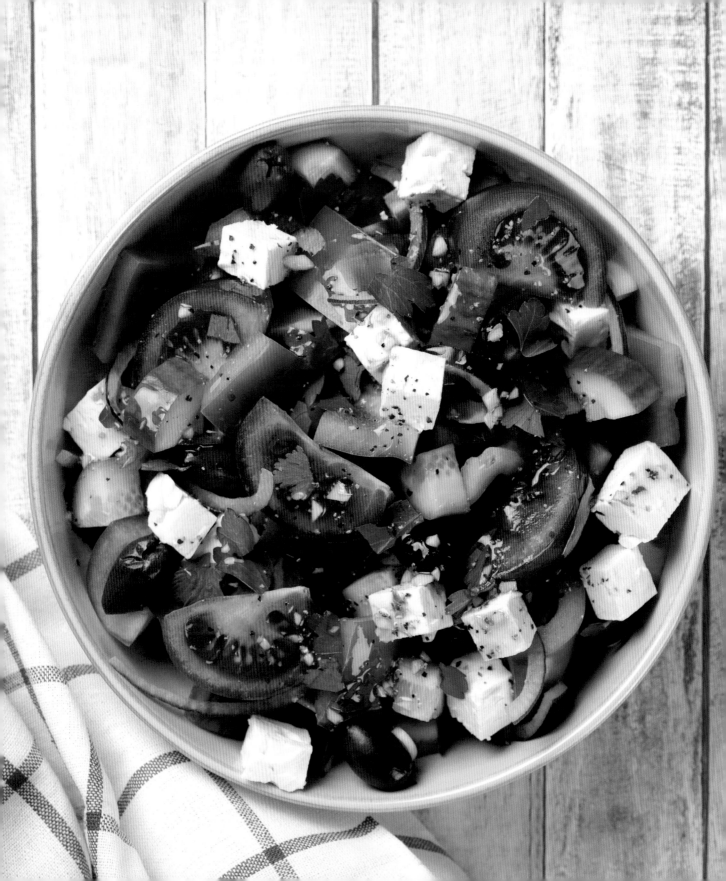

salads *and* sides

PER SERVING

233 calories
21g **total fat**
7g **carbs**
6g **net carbs**
1g **dietary fiber**
8g **protein**

Greek Salad

makes 6 servings

Salad

3 medium tomatoes, cut into 8 wedges each

1 green bell pepper, cut into 1-inch pieces

½ English cucumber (8 to 10 inches), quartered lengthwise and sliced crosswise

½ red onion, thinly sliced

½ cup pitted kalamata olives

1 package (8 ounces) feta cheese, cut into ½-inch cubes

Dressing

6 tablespoons extra virgin olive oil

3 tablespoons red wine vinegar

1 to 2 cloves garlic, minced

¾ teaspoon dried oregano

¾ teaspoon salt

¼ teaspoon black pepper

1. Combine tomatoes, bell pepper, cucumber, onion and olives in large bowl. Top with feta.

2. For dressing, whisk oil, vinegar, garlic, oregano, salt and pepper in medium bowl until well blended. Pour over salad; stir gently to coat.

Mediterranean Shrimp and Feta Salad

makes 4 servings

1 pound large raw shrimp, unpeeled

1 teaspoon salt

4 cups (6 ounces) baby spinach

2 large plum tomatoes, cored and chopped

2 ounces feta cheese, crumbled

¼ cup chopped green onions

¼ cup coarsely chopped pitted kalamata olives

1 tablespoon minced fresh oregano or basil

3 tablespoons extra virgin olive oil

1 tablespoon red wine vinegar

1 tablespoon small capers

½ teaspoon freshly ground black pepper

1. Place shrimp in large saucepan with 1 quart of water. Add salt; bring to simmer over medium-high heat. Simmer 8 to 10 minutes or until shrimp are pink and opaque. Drain and set aside until cool enough to handle. Peel and cut into bite-size pieces.

2. Place shrimp in large serving bowl. Add spinach, tomatoes, feta, green onions, olives and oregano. Combine oil, vinegar, capers and pepper in small bowl; mix well. Pour over salad and toss gently.

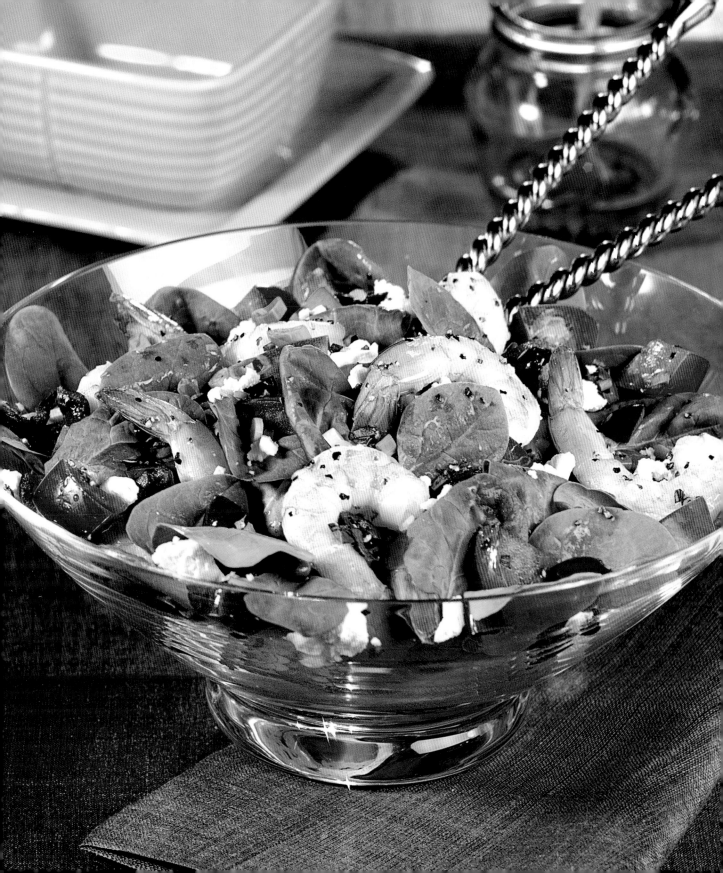

Kale with Caramelized Garlic

makes 6 servings

1½ pounds fresh kale, tough stems removed and discarded, leaves thinly sliced (16 cups)

2 cups water

1 tablespoon olive oil

8 cloves garlic, thinly sliced

1 teaspoon red wine vinegar

¼ teaspoon salt

⅛ to ¼ teaspoon red pepper flakes

1. Place kale and water in large saucepan; bring to a boil over medium-high heat. Cover and cook 6 to 8 minutes or until kale is tender but still bright green. Drain in colander.

2. Meanwhile, heat oil in large nonstick skillet over medium heat. Add garlic; cook and stir 4 minutes or until garlic is golden brown, being careful not to allow garlic to burn. Add kale, vinegar, salt and red pepper flakes; cook and stir until heated through.

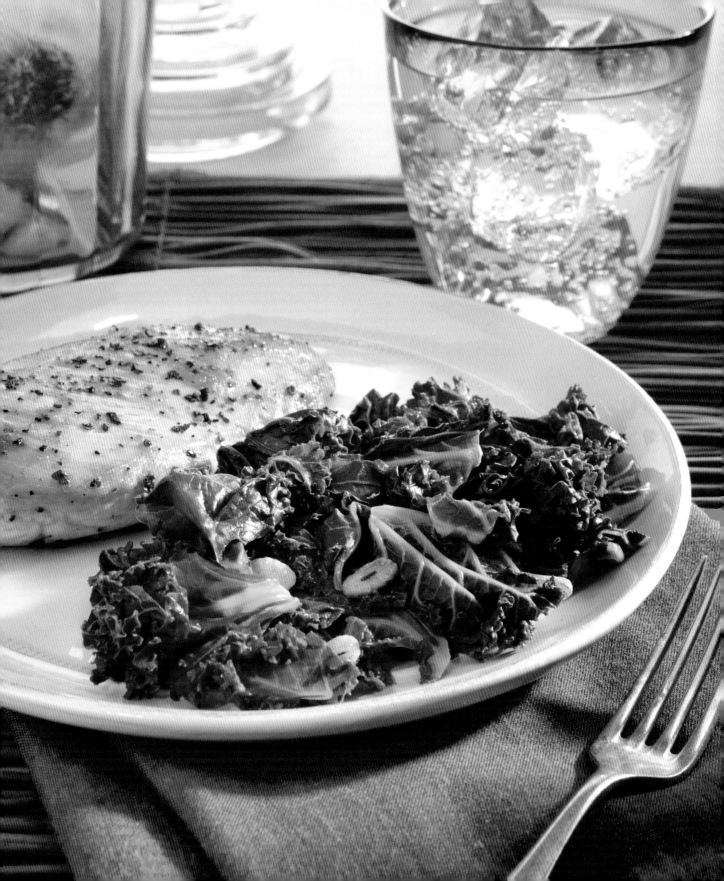

Shrimp, Feta and Tomato Salad

makes 4 servings

PER SERVING

137 calories
6g total fat
4g carbs
3g net carbs
1g dietary fiber
16g protein

8 ounces cooked medium shrimp, peeled and deveined

1 pint (2 cups) cherry tomatoes, halved (or whole small yellow pear tomatoes)

¼ cup thinly sliced fresh basil

1 tablespoon olive oil

1 tablespoon white wine vinegar

¼ teaspoon black pepper

8 large Boston lettuce leaves

½ cup crumbled feta cheese

Combine shrimp, tomatoes, basil, oil, vinegar and pepper in medium bowl; mix well. Serve over lettuce and top with cheese.

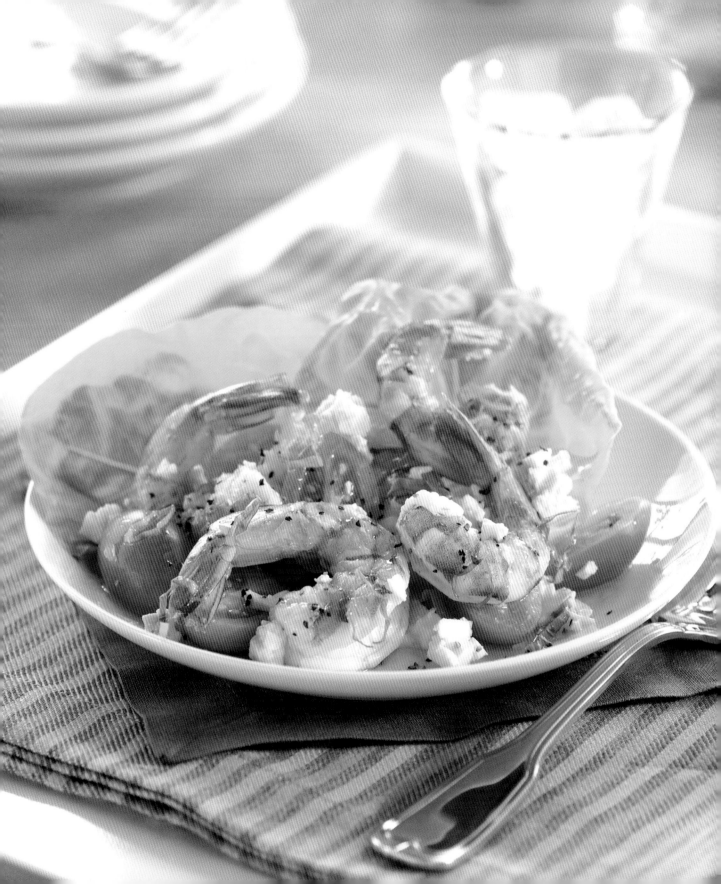

Cheese Soufflé

makes 4 servings

¼ cup (½ stick) butter

¼ cup almond flour

1½ cups milk, warmed to room temperature

¼ teaspoon salt

¼ teaspoon ground red pepper

⅛ teaspoon black pepper

6 eggs, separated

1 cup (4 ounces) shredded Cheddar cheese

Pinch cream of tartar (optional)

1. Preheat oven to 375°F. Grease four 2-cup soufflé dishes or one 2-quart soufflé dish.

2. Melt butter in large saucepan over medium-low heat. Add almond flour; whisk 2 minutes or until mixture just begins to color. Gradually whisk in milk. Add salt, red pepper and black pepper; whisk until mixture comes to a boil and thickens. Remove from heat. Stir in egg yolks, one at a time, and cheese.

3. Beat egg whites and cream of tartar in large bowl with electric mixer at high speed until stiff peaks form.

4. Gently fold egg whites into cheese mixture until almost combined. (Some streaks of white should remain.) Transfer mixture to prepared dishes.

5. Bake small soufflés about 20 minutes (30 to 40 minutes for large soufflé) or until puffed and browned and skewer inserted into center comes out moist but clean. Serve immediately.

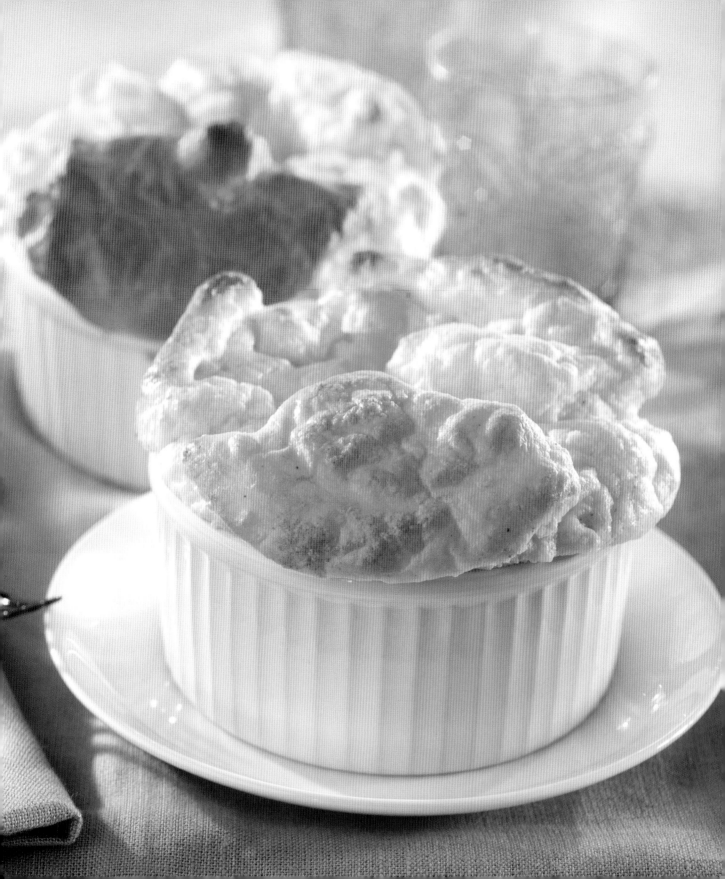

Scallop and Spinach Salad

makes 4 servings

1 package (10 ounces) fresh spinach leaves, washed, stemmed and torn

3 thin slices red onion, halved and separated

12 ounces sea scallops

⅛ teaspoon ground red pepper

⅛ teaspoon paprika

½ cup Italian salad dressing

¼ cup crumbled blue cheese

2 tablespoons toasted walnuts

1. Pat spinach dry; place in large bowl with onion. Cover; set aside.

2. Rinse scallops. Cut in half horizontally (to make 2 thin rounds); pat dry. Sprinkle top sides lightly with red pepper and paprika.

3. Spray large nonstick skillet with nonstick cooking spray; heat over high heat until very hot. Add half of scallops, seasoned sides down, in single layer, placing ½ inch or more apart. Cook 2 minutes or until browned on bottom. Turn scallops; cook 1 to 2 minutes or until opaque in center. Transfer to plate; cover to keep warm. Wipe skillet clean; repeat with remaining scallops.

4. Place dressing in small saucepan; bring to a boil over high heat. Pour dressing over spinach and onion; toss to coat. Divide among 4 plates. Place scallops on top of spinach; sprinkle with cheese and walnuts.

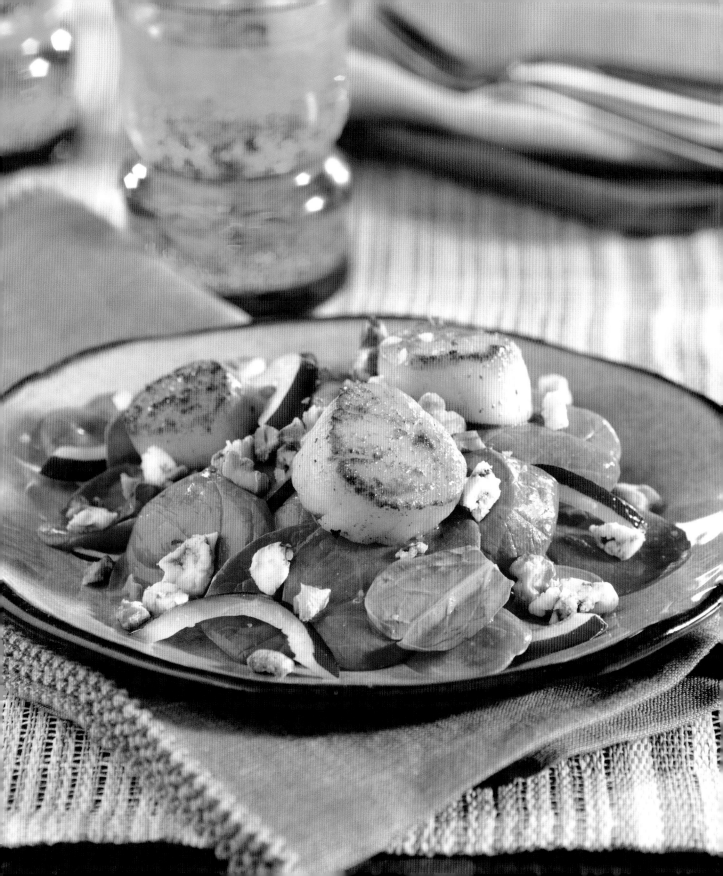

Broccoli Italian Style

makes 4 servings

1¼   **pounds fresh broccoli**

2   **tablespoons lemon juice**

1   **teaspoon extra virgin olive oil**

1   **clove garlic, minced**

1   **teaspoon chopped fresh Italian parsley**

Dash black pepper

1. Trim broccoli, discarding tough stems. Cut broccoli into florets with 2-inch stems. Peel remaining stems; cut into ½-inch slices.

2. Bring 1 quart water to a boil in large saucepan over medium-high heat. Add broccoli; return to a boil. Cook 3 to 5 minutes or until broccoli is tender. Drain; transfer to serving dish.

3. Combine lemon juice, oil, garlic, parsley and pepper in small bowl. Pour over broccoli; toss to coat. Cover and let stand 1 hour before serving to allow flavors to blend. Serve at room temperature.

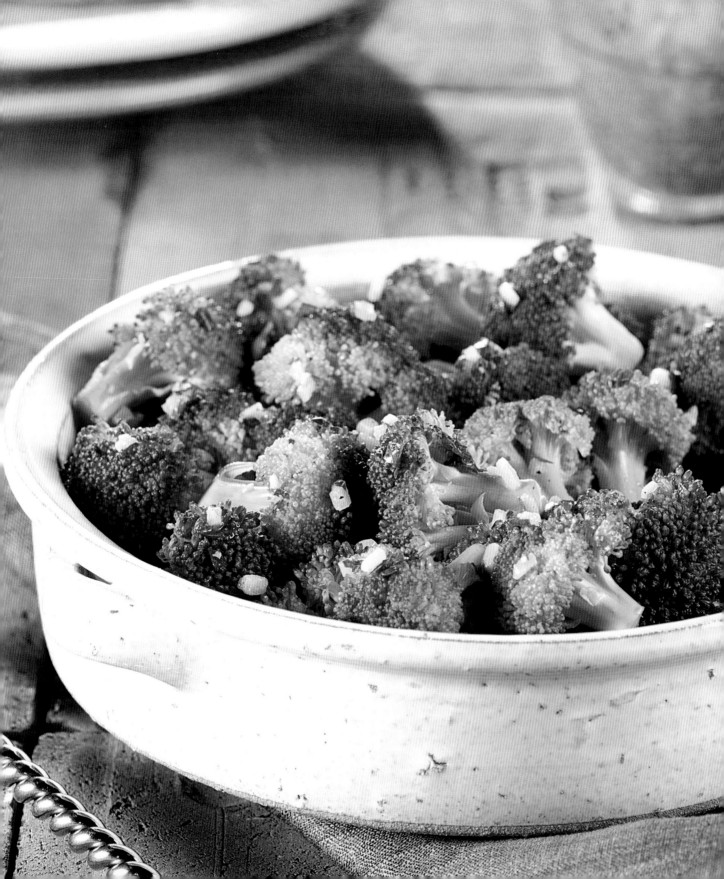

Steakhouse Chopped Salad

makes 10 servings (20 cups)

Dressing

- ⅓ cup white balsamic vinegar
- ¼ cup Dijon mustard
- 1 package (about 2 tablespoons) Italian salad dressing mix
- ⅔ cup extra virgin olive oil

Salad

- 1 medium head iceberg lettuce, chopped
- 1 medium head romaine lettuce, chopped
- 1 can (about 14 ounces) artichoke hearts, quartered lengthwise then sliced crosswise
- 1 large avocado, diced
- 1½ cups crumbled blue cheese
- 2 hard-cooked eggs, chopped
- 1 ripe tomato, chopped
- ½ small red onion, finely chopped
- 12 slices bacon, crisp-cooked and crumbled

1. For dressing, whisk vinegar, mustard and dressing mix in small bowl. Slowly add oil, whisking until well blended. Set aside until ready to use. (Dressing can be made up to 1 week in advance; refrigerate in jar with tight-fitting lid.)

2. For salad, combine lettuce, artichokes, avocado, cheese, eggs, tomato, onion and bacon in large bowl. Add dressing; toss to coat.

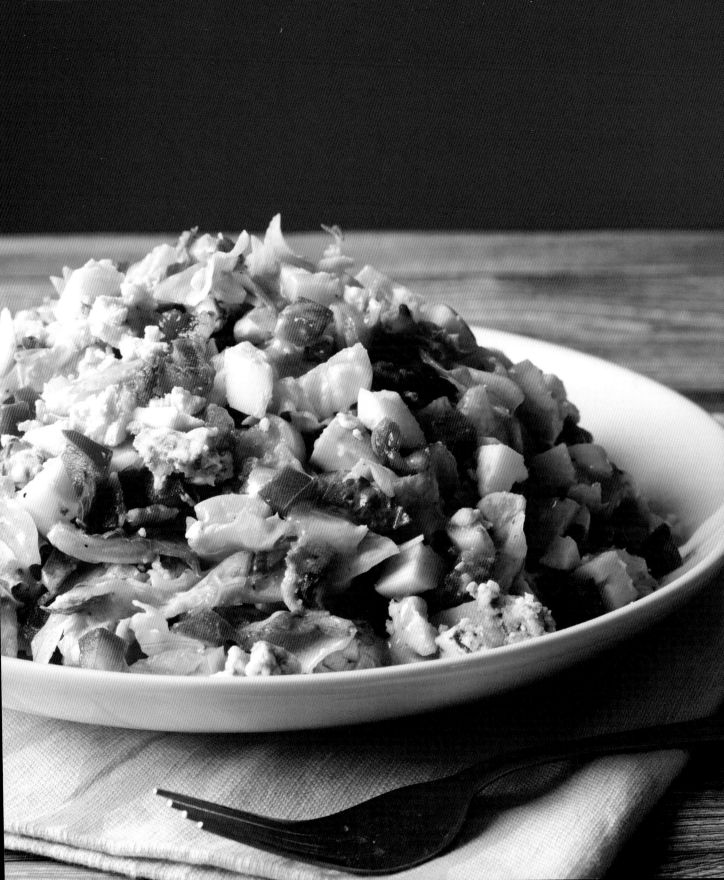

Mashed Cauliflower

makes 6 servings

PER SERVING

54 **calories**
2g **total fat**
7g **carbs**
4g **net carbs**
3g **dietary fiber**
3g **protein**

2 heads cauliflower (to equal 8 cups florets)

1 tablespoon butter

1 tablespoon half-and-half or whipping cream

   Salt

1. Break cauliflower into equal-size florets. Place in large saucepan in about 2 inches of water. Simmer over medium heat 20 to 25 minutes, or until cauliflower is very tender and falling apart. (Check occasionally to make sure there is enough water to prevent burning; add water if necessary.) Drain well.

2. Place cooked cauliflower in food processor or blender. Process until almost smooth. Add butter. Process until smooth, adding half-and-half as needed to reach desired consistency. Season with salt to taste.

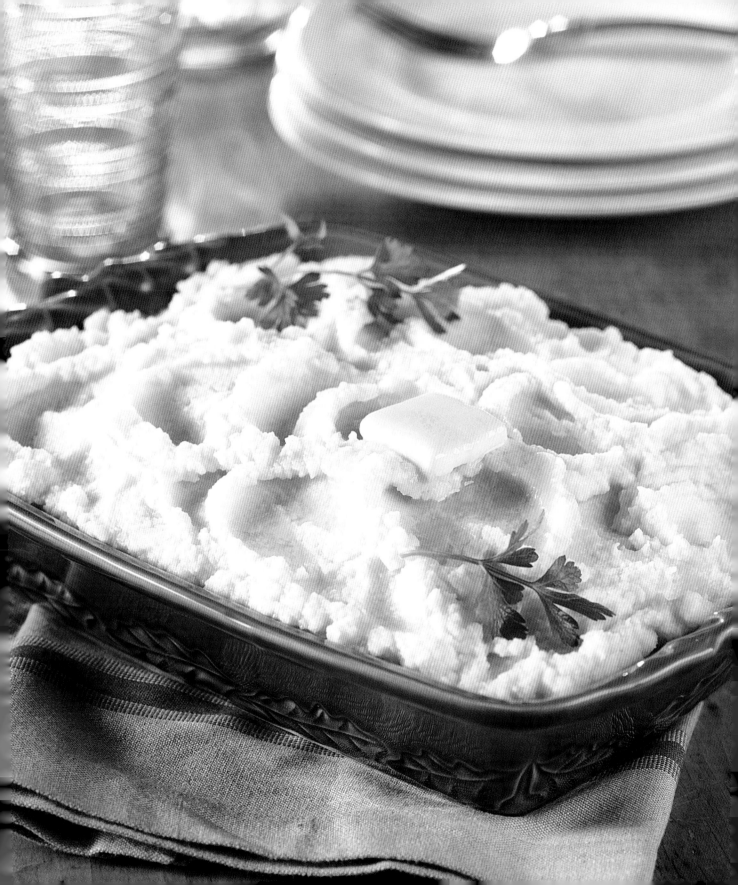

Green Goddess Cobb Salad

makes 4 servings

Pickled Onions

- 1 cup thinly sliced red onion
- ½ cup white wine vinegar
- ¼ cup water
- 1 teaspoon salt

Dressing

- 1 cup mayonnaise
- 1 cup fresh Italian parsley leaves
- 1 cup baby arugula
- ¼ cup extra virgin olive oil
- 3 tablespoons lemon juice
- 3 tablespoons minced fresh chives
- 2 tablespoons fresh tarragon leaves
- 1 clove garlic, minced
- 1 teaspoon Dijon mustard
- ½ teaspoon salt
- ⅛ teaspoon black pepper

Salad

- 4 eggs
- 4 cups Italian salad blend (romaine and radicchio)
- 2 cups chopped stemmed kale
- 2 cups baby arugula
- 2 avocados, sliced and halved
- 2 tomatoes, cut into wedges
- 2 cups cooked chicken strips
- 1 cup chopped crisp-cooked bacon

1. For pickled onions, combine onion, vinegar, ¼ cup water and 1 teaspoon salt in large glass jar. Seal jar; shake well. Refrigerate at least 1 hour or up to 1 week.

2. For dressing, combine mayonnaise, parsley, 1 cup arugula, oil, lemon juice, chives, tarragon, garlic, mustard, ½ teaspoon salt and pepper in blender or food processor; blend until smooth, stopping to scrape down side once or twice. Transfer to jar; refrigerate until ready to use. Just before serving, thin dressing with 1 to 2 tablespoons water, if necessary, to reach desired consistency.

3. Fill medium saucepan with water; bring to a boil over high heat. Carefully lower eggs into water. Reduce heat to medium; boil gently 12 minutes. Drain eggs; add cold water and ice cubes to saucepan to cool eggs. When eggs are cool enough to handle, peel and cut in half lengthwise.

4. For salad, combine salad blend, kale, 2 cups arugula and pickled onions in large bowl; divide among 4 individual serving bowls. Top each salad with avocados, tomatoes, chicken, bacon and two egg halves. Top with ¼ cup dressing; toss to coat.

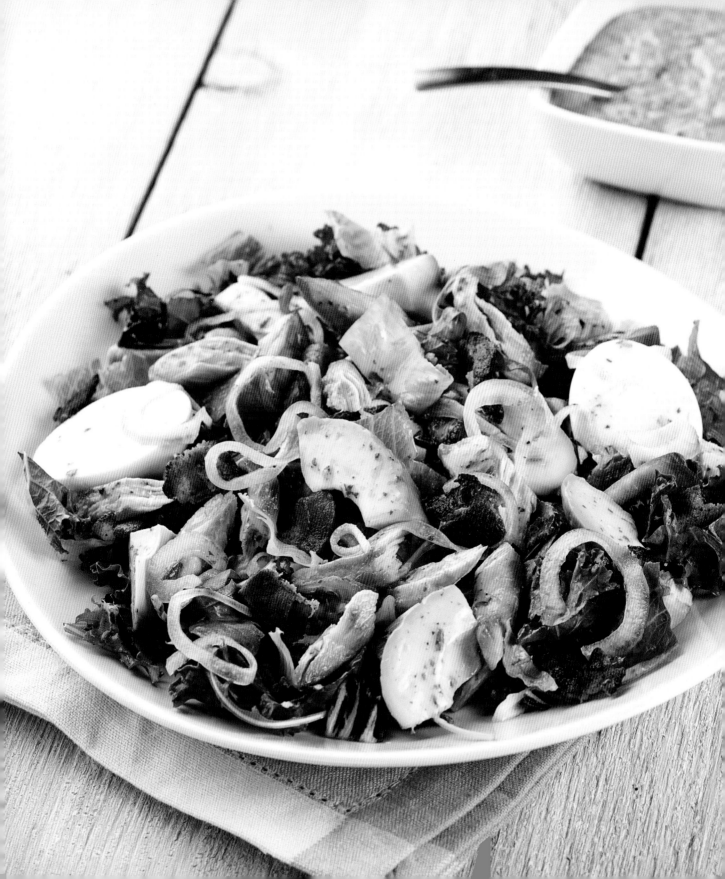

Asparagus with Creamy Garlic Dressing

makes 4 servings

2 tablespoons sour cream

1 tablespoon buttermilk or whipping cream

1 teaspoon grated lemon peel

1 clove garlic, minced

Salt and black pepper

24 asparagus spears, trimmed and diagonally sliced into 1-inch pieces

1. Whisk sour cream, buttermilk, lemon peel and garlic in small bowl. Season with salt and pepper.

2. Place asparagus in large skillet; add enough water to just cover asparagus and season with salt. Bring to a boil over high heat. Reduce heat to a simmer; cook 3 to 5 minutes or until asparagus is crisp-tender. Drain and rinse under cold water to stop cooking. Place in serving bowl. Add dressing; stir until well coated.

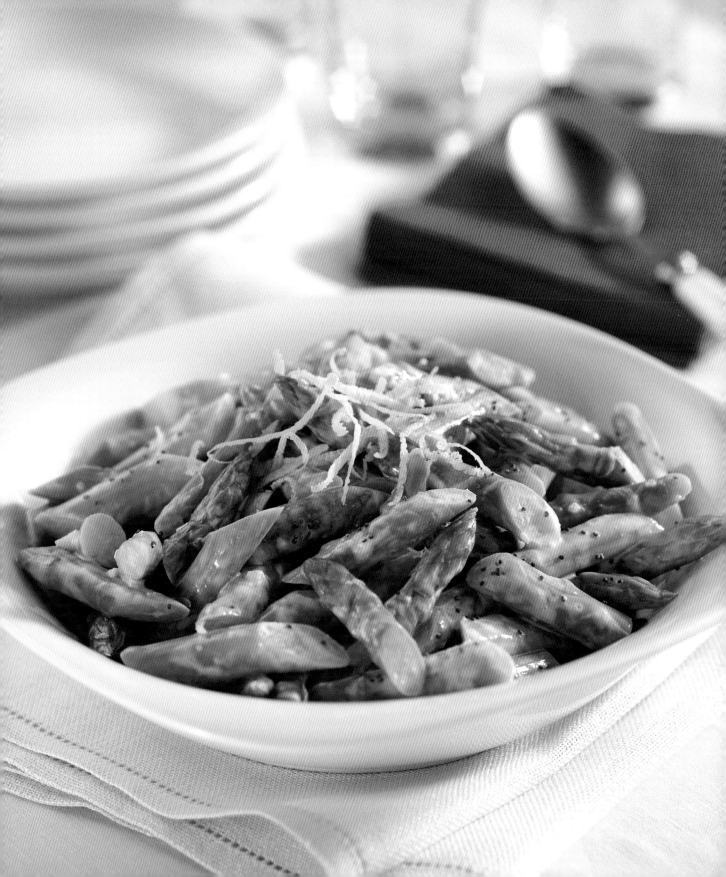

Garbage Salad

makes 4 servings

PER SERVING

420 calories
35g total fat
10g carbs
7g net carbs
3g dietary fiber
19g protein

Dressing

- ⅓ cup red wine vinegar
- 2 cloves garlic, minced
- 1 teaspoon Italian seasoning
- ¼ teaspoon salt
- ¼ teaspoon black pepper
- ⅓ cup olive oil

Salad

- 1 package (5 ounces) spring mix
- 5 leaves romaine lettuce, chopped
- 1 small cucumber, diced
- 2 small plum tomatoes, diced
- ½ red onion, thinly sliced
- ¼ cup pitted kalamata olives
- 4 radishes, thinly sliced
- 4 ounces thinly sliced Genoa salami, cut into ¼-inch strips
- 4 ounces provolone cheese, cut into ¼-inch strips
- ¼ cup grated Parmesan cheese

1. For dressing, whisk vinegar, garlic, Italian seasoning, salt and pepper in small bowl until blended. Slowly whisk in oil in thin steady stream until well blended.

2. Combine spring mix, romaine, cucumber, tomatoes, onion, olives and radishes in large bowl. Add half of dressing; toss gently to coat. Top with salami and provolone; sprinkle with Parmesan. Serve with remaining dressing.

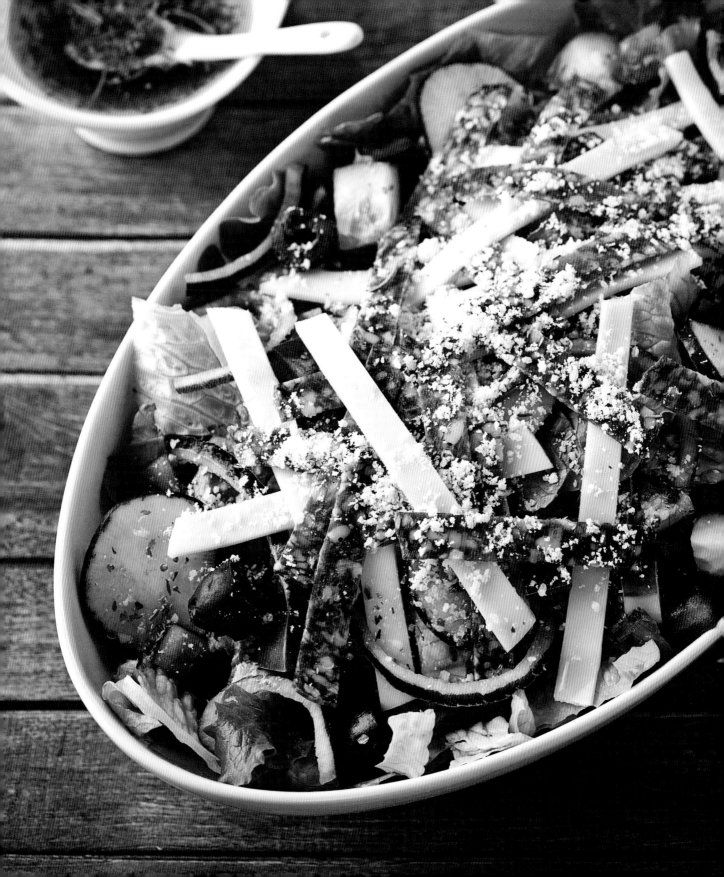

Smoky Kale Chiffonade

makes 4 servings

¾ **pound fresh young kale or mustard greens**

3 **slices bacon**

2 **tablespoons crumbled blue cheese**

1. Rinse kale well in large bowl of warm water; drain in colander. Discard any discolored leaves; trim away tough stem ends. To prepare chiffonade, stack leaves and roll up from long end. Slice crosswise into ½-inch slices; separate into strips. Set aside.

2. Cook bacon in medium skillet over medium heat until crisp. Remove bacon to paper towel. Drain all but 1 tablespoon drippings.

3. Add kale to drippings in skillet. Cook and stir over medium-high heat 2 to 3 minutes until wilted and tender (older leaves may take slightly longer).

4. Crumble bacon; add to kale with cheese. Toss gently to blend. Transfer to warm serving dish. Serve immediately.

Note: "Chiffonade" in French literally means "made of rags." In cooking, it means "cut into thin strips."

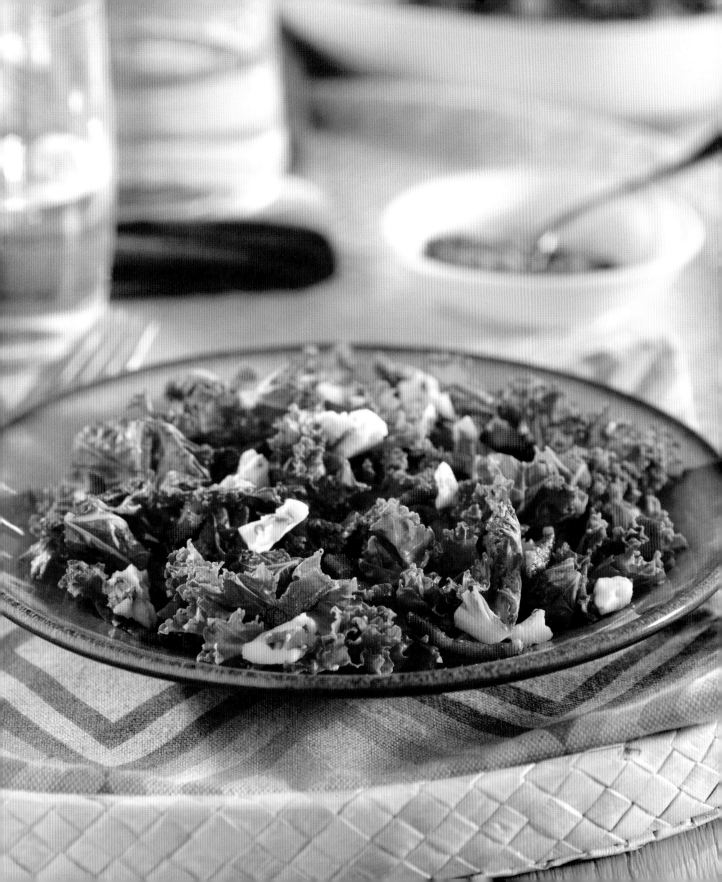

Layered Caprese Salad

makes 4 servings

PER SERVING

94 calories
5g total fat
9g carbs
6g net carbs
3g dietary fiber
5g protein

2 tablespoons extra virgin olive oil

2 teaspoons balsamic vinegar

2 cloves garlic, minced

Salt and black pepper

½ small red onion, thinly sliced

3 medium tomatoes, sliced

½ cup (2 ounces) shredded mozzarella cheese

2 tablespoons chopped fresh parsley

2 tablespoons shredded fresh basil

1. Whisk oil, vinegar, garlic, salt and pepper in small bowl until well blended.

2. Spread half of onion in serving dish. Layer with half of tomatoes and sprinkle with half of cheese, parsley and basil. Drizzle with half of dressing. Repeat layers of onions, tomatoes, herbs and dressing. Serve at room temperature or cover and refrigerate 1 hour.

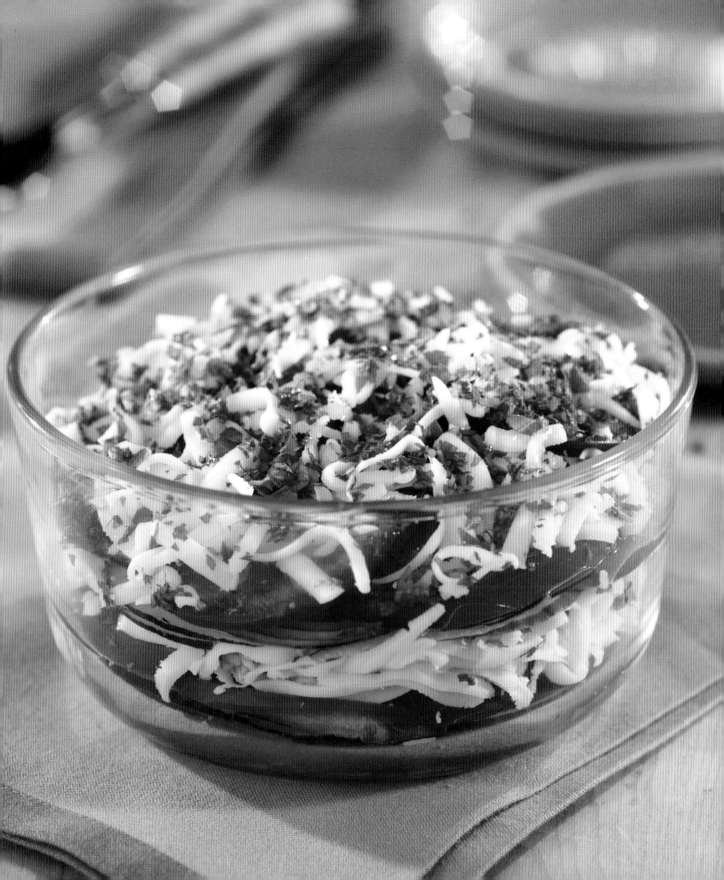

Taco Salad Supreme

makes 4 servings

PER SERVING

584 calories
47g total fat
11g carbs
6g net carbs
5g dietary fiber
30g protein

1 pound ground beef

½ cup chopped onion

2 cloves garlic, minced

1 teaspoon ground cumin

1 teaspoon chili powder

½ teaspoon salt

½ cup salsa, divided

6 cups packed torn or sliced romaine lettuce

1 large tomato, chopped

1 cup (4 ounces) shredded Mexican cheese blend or taco cheese, divided

2 tablespoons canola oil

1 ripe avocado, diced

¼ cup sour cream

1. Brown beef and onion in large skillet over medium-high heat 6 to 8 minutes, stirring to break up meat. Drain fat. Add garlic, cumin, chili powder and salt; cook 1 minute, stirring frequently. Stir in ¼ cup salsa; cook and stir 1 minute. Remove from heat.

2. Combine lettuce, tomato, ½ cup cheese, remaining ¼ cup salsa and oil in large bowl. Divide salad among 4 serving plates. Spoon meat mixture evenly over salads; top with remaining ½ cup cheese, avocado and sour cream.

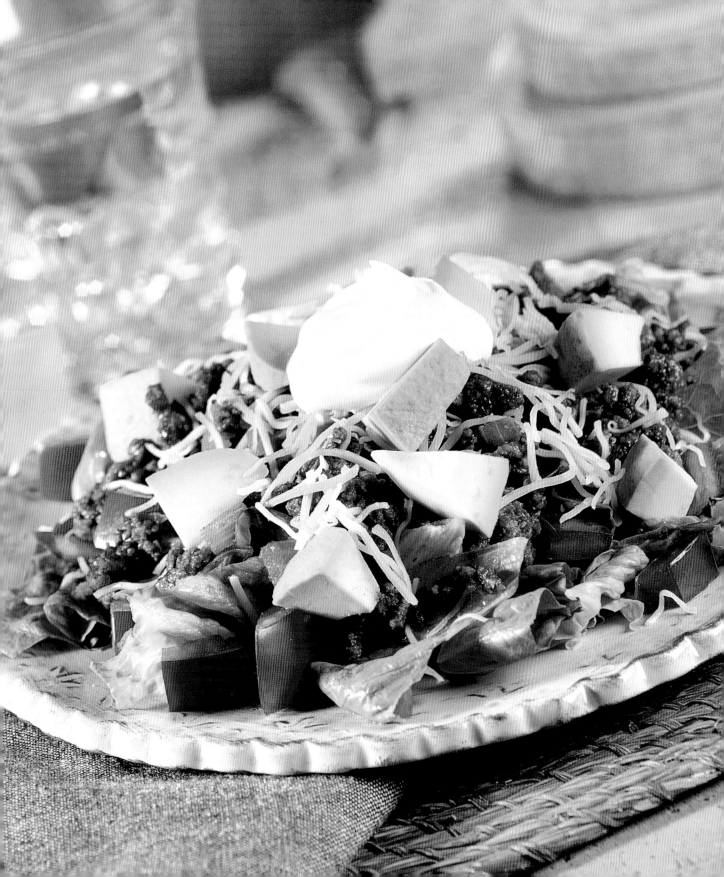

Red Cabbage with Bacon and Mushrooms

makes 6 servings

5 slices thick-cut bacon, chopped (about 8 ounces)

1 onion, chopped

1 package (8 ounces) cremini mushrooms, chopped (½-inch pieces)

¾ teaspoon dried thyme

½ medium red cabbage, cut into wedges, cored and then cut crosswise into ¼-inch slices (about 7 cups)

¾ teaspoon salt

¼ teaspoon black pepper

⅔ cup chicken broth

3 tablespoons cider vinegar

¼ cup chopped walnuts, toasted*

3 tablespoons chopped fresh parsley

To toast walnuts, cook in small skillet over medium heat 4 to 5 minutes or until lightly browned, stirring frequently.

1. Cook bacon in large saucepan or skillet over medium-high heat until crisp. Remove to paper towel-lined plate.

2. Add onion to saucepan; cook and stir 5 minutes or until softened. Add mushrooms and thyme; cook about 6 minutes or until mushrooms begin to brown, stirring occasionally. Add cabbage, ¾ teaspoon salt and ¼ teaspoon pepper; cook about 7 minutes or until cabbage has wilted.

3. Stir in broth, vinegar and half of bacon; bring to a boil. Reduce heat to low; cook, uncovered, 15 to 20 minutes or until cabbage is tender.

4. Stir in walnuts and parsley; season with additional salt and pepper, if desired. Sprinkle with remaining bacon.

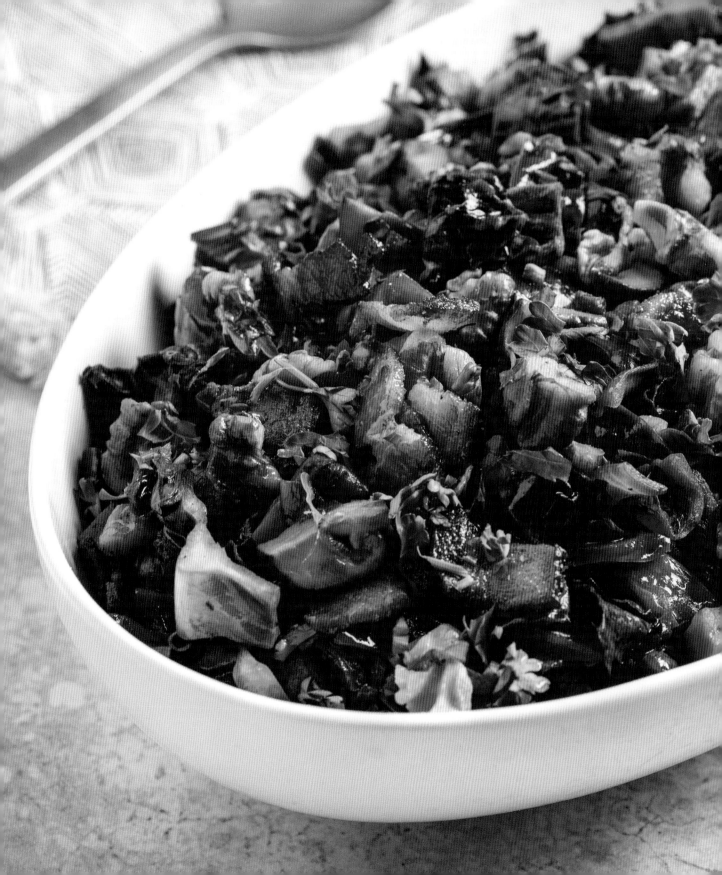

Crab Spinach Salad with Tarragon Dressing

makes 4 servings

- 12 ounces coarsely flaked cooked crabmeat *or* 2 packages (6 ounces each) frozen crabmeat, thawed and drained
- 1 cup chopped tomatoes
- 1 cup sliced cucumber
- ⅓ cup sliced red onion
- ¼ cup mayonnaise
- ¼ cup sour cream
- ¼ cup chopped fresh parsley
- 2 tablespoons milk
- 2 teaspoons chopped fresh tarragon *or* ½ teaspoon dried tarragon
- 1 clove garlic, minced
- ¼ teaspoon hot pepper sauce
- 8 cups fresh spinach

1. Combine crabmeat, tomatoes, cucumber and onion in medium bowl. Combine mayonnaise, sour cream, parsley, milk, tarragon, garlic and hot pepper sauce in small bowl.

2. Line 4 salad plates with spinach. Place crabmeat mixture on spinach; drizzle with dressing.

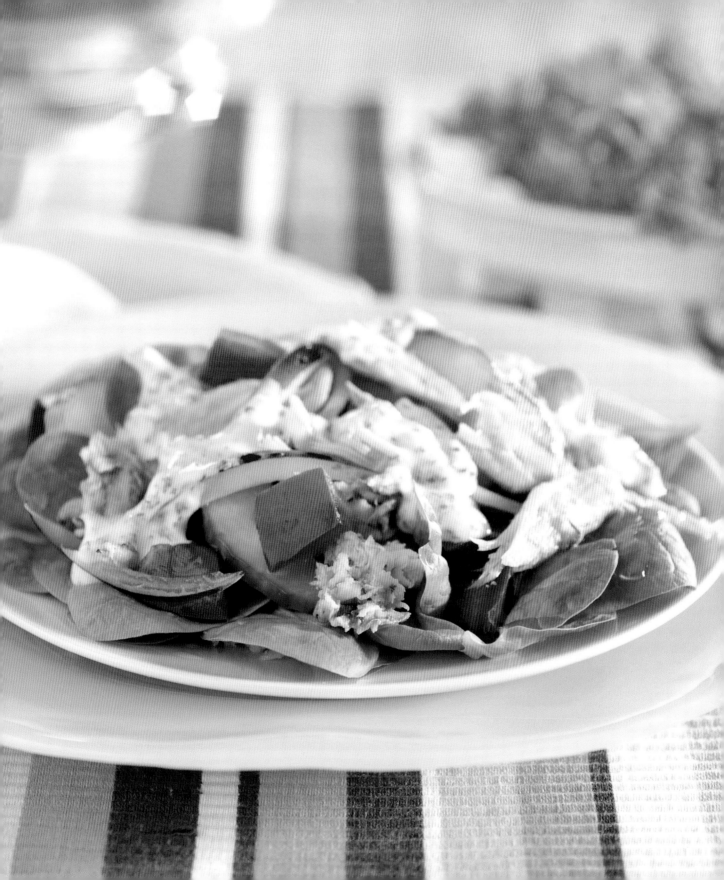

Roasted Cauliflower

makes 4 servings (about ¾ cup per serving)

5 cups cauliflower florets

1 tablespoon extra virgin olive oil

¾ teaspoon Italian seasoning

½ teaspoon garlic powder

¼ teaspoon salt

⅛ teaspoon black pepper

1. Preheat oven to 425°F. Spray baking sheet with nonstick cooking spray.

2. Place cauliflower on prepared baking sheet. Drizzle with oil. Sprinkle evenly with Italian seasoning, garlic powder, salt and pepper. Gently toss; arrange in single layer.

3. Bake 20 minutes or until tender, turning once.

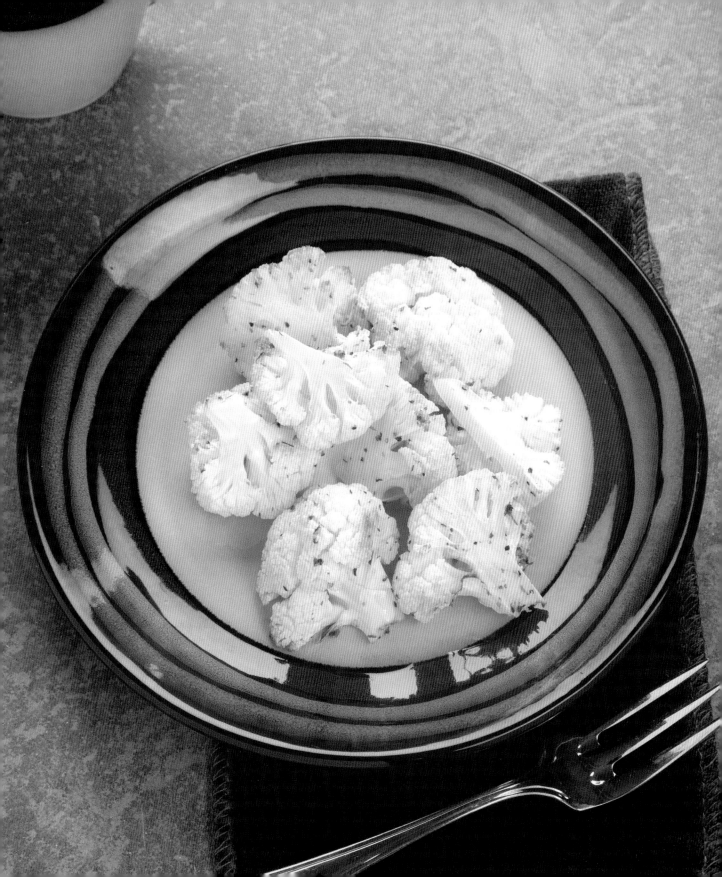

Herbed Zucchini Ribbons

makes 4 servings

PER SERVING

180 **calories**
7g **total fat**
3g **carbs**
2g **net carbs**
1g **dietary fiber**
1g **protein**

- 3 small zucchini (about ¾ pound total)
- 2 tablespoons olive oil
- 1 tablespoon white wine vinegar
- 2 teaspoons chopped fresh basil *or* ½ teaspoon dried basil
- ½ teaspoon red pepper flakes
- ¼ teaspoon ground coriander
- Salt and black pepper

1. To make zucchini ribbons, cut tip and stem ends from zucchini with paring knife. Using vegetable peeler, begin at stem end and make continuous ribbons down length of each zucchini.

2. To steam zucchini ribbons, place steamer basket in large saucepan; add 1 inch of water. (Water should not touch bottom of basket.) Place zucchini ribbons in steamer basket; cover. Bring to a boil over high heat. When pan begins to steam, check zucchini for doneness. (It should be crisp-tender.) Transfer zucchini to warm serving dish with slotted spatula or tongs.

3. Whisk oil, vinegar, basil, red pepper flakes and coriander in small bowl until well blended.

4. Pour dressing mixture over zucchini ribbons; toss gently to coat. Season with salt and black pepper. Serve immediately or refrigerate up to 2 days.

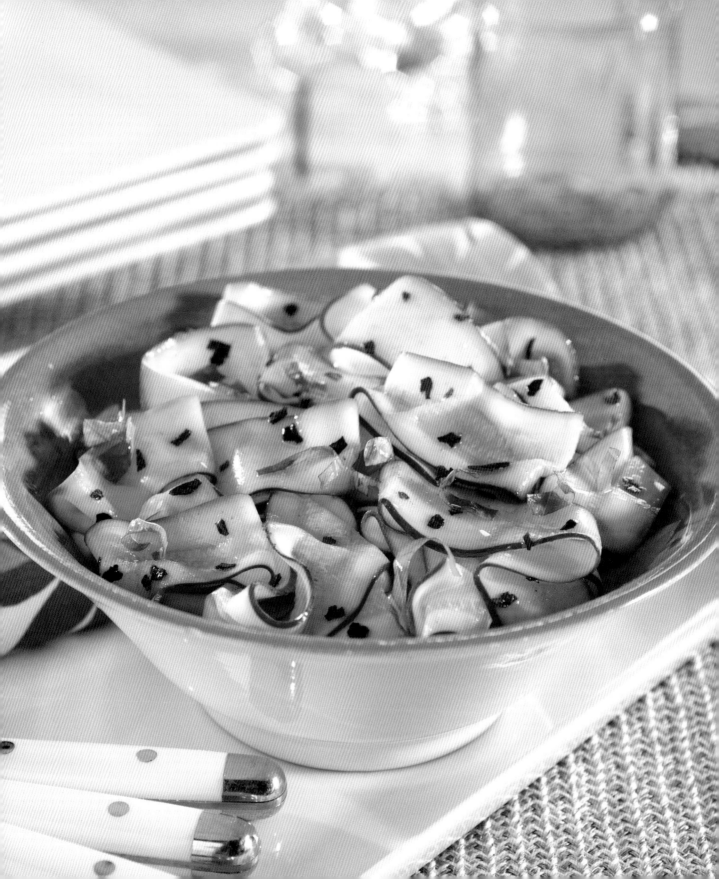

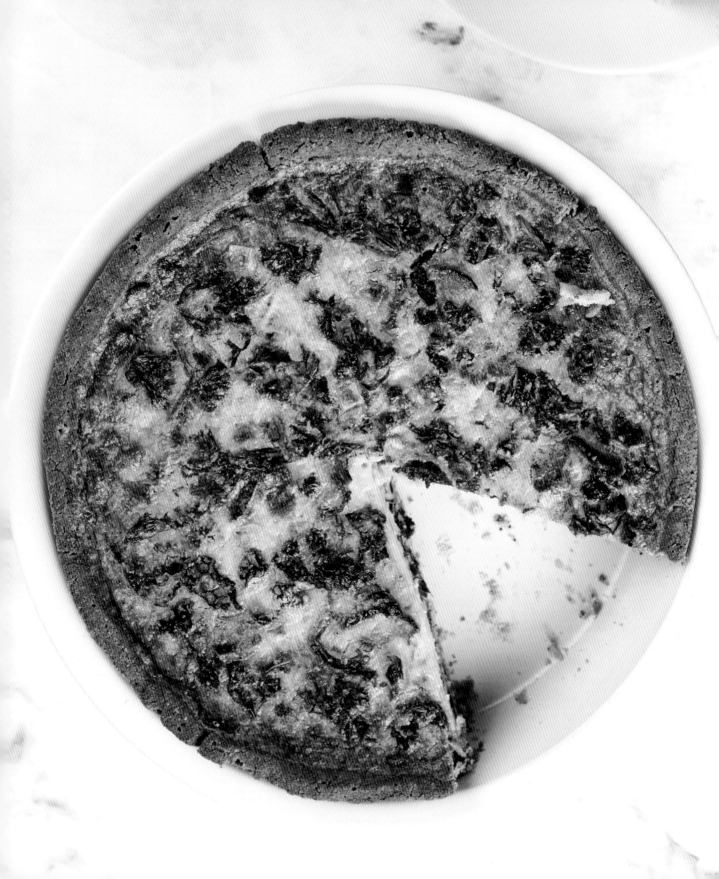

breakfast and egg dishes

Bacon-Kale Quiche

makes 6 servings

Crust

- ¾ cup coconut flour
- ¾ cup almond flour
- ¼ teaspoon salt
- 2 eggs
- 6 tablespoons coconut oil or butter, melted

Filling

- 8 eggs
- ½ cup whipping cream
- 1 package (12 ounces) bacon
- 1 cup chopped onion
- 3 cups tightly packed chopped stemmed kale
- ½ cup finely shredded Parmesan cheese
- ¼ cup finely chopped sun-dried tomatoes

1. Preheat oven to 375°F. Combine coconut flour, almond flour and salt in medium bowl. Stir in 2 eggs and coconut oil until well blended. Press onto bottom and up side of deep dish pie plate. Bake 5 minutes.

2. Whisk eggs and cream in large bowl until well blended. Cook bacon in large skillet until crisp. Drain on paper towels; chop when cool enough to handle. Add onion and kale to drippings in skillet; cook and stir over medium heat about 5 minutes or until onion is golden and kale is wilted. Add vegetables and drippings to eggs; mix well. Stir in cheese, tomatoes and bacon. Pour into prepared crust.

3. Bake 40 minutes or until quiche is puffed and knife inserted into center comes out clean, covering edges of crust with foil after 20 minutes to prevent overbrowning. Let stand 20 minutes before cutting.

Deep South Ham and Redeye Gravy

makes 4 servings

1 tablespoon butter

1 ham steak (about 1⅓ pounds)

1 cup strong coffee

¼ teaspoon hot pepper sauce

1. Heat large skillet over medium-high heat until hot. Add butter; tilt skillet to coat bottom. Add ham steak; cook 3 minutes. Turn; cook 2 minutes longer or until lightly browned. Remove ham to serving platter; keep warm.

2. Add coffee and hot pepper sauce to same skillet. Bring to a boil over high heat; boil 2 to 3 minutes or until liquid is reduced to ¼ cup, scraping up any brown bits from bottom of skillet. Serve gravy over ham.

Serving Suggestion: Serve ham steak with sautéed greens and poached eggs.

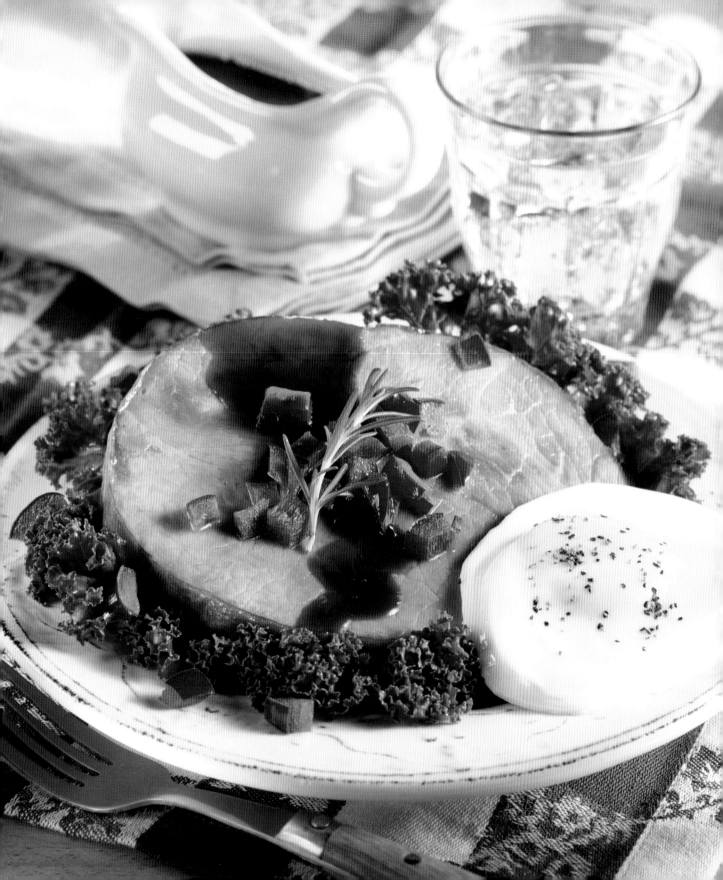

Pepperoni Frittata

makes 4 servings

PER SERVING

170 calories
6g total fat
9g carbs
8g net carbs
1g dietary fiber
22g protein

2 cups liquid egg substitute *or* 8 eggs, lightly beaten

⅓ cup evaporated milk

1 ounce turkey pepperoni slices, chopped (about 16 slices)

¼ cup finely chopped green onions

½ teaspoon dried rosemary

½ teaspoon dried basil

⅛ teaspoon salt

⅛ teaspoon black pepper

2 medium plum tomatoes, thinly sliced

¾ cup (3 ounces) shredded mozzarella cheese

Thinly sliced fresh basil (optional)

1. Preheat broiler.

2. Combine egg substitute, milk, pepperoni, green onions, rosemary, basil, salt and pepper in medium bowl.

3. Spray medium ovenproof nonstick skillet with nonstick cooking spray; heat over medium heat. Add egg mixture; reduce heat to medium-low. Cook 8 to 10 minutes or until edge is set (center will still be wet).

4. Place skillet under broiler 4 inches away from heat source; broil 1 minute or until eggs are set.

5. Arrange tomatoes on top of frittata; sprinkle with cheese. Broil 1 minute or until cheese is melted. Let stand 5 minutes before serving. Garnish with basil.

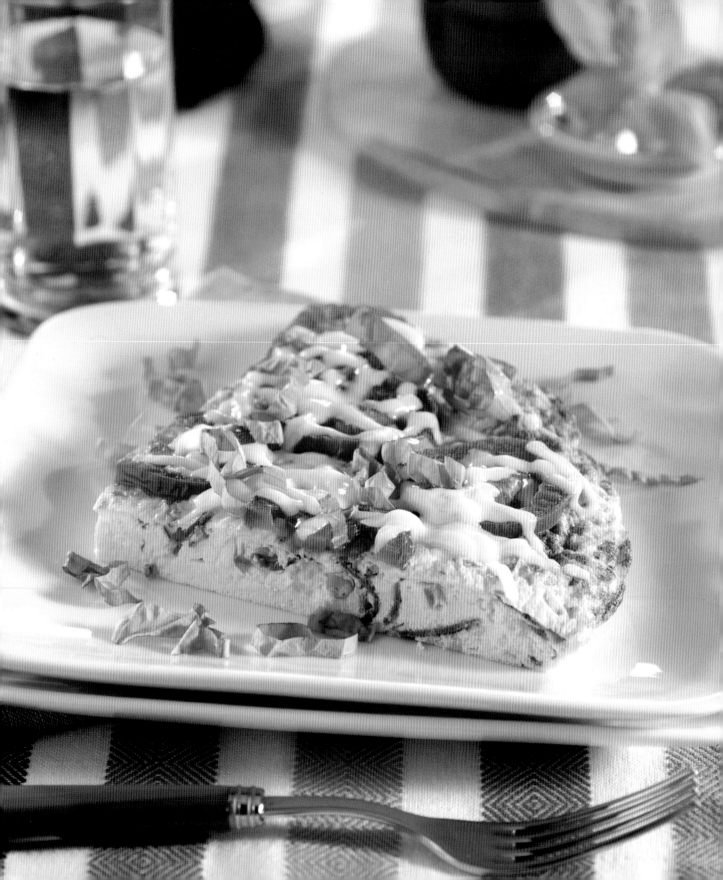

Cheddar, Broccoli and Mushroom Quiche

makes 4 servings

PER SERVING

157 calories
6g total fat
8g carbs
6g net carbs
2g dietary fiber
19g protein

- **6 ounces sliced mushrooms**
- **1½ cups small broccoli florets (½-inch pieces)**
- **1½ cups liquid egg substitute *or* 6 eggs, beaten**
- **⅓ cup milk**
- **½ teaspoon salt**
- **¼ teaspoon dried thyme**
- **⅛ teaspoon ground red pepper**
- **½ cup finely chopped green onions**
- **1 cup (4 ounces) shredded sharp Cheddar cheese, divided**

1. Preheat oven to 350°F. Spray 9-inch deep-dish glass pie plate with nonstick cooking spray.

2. Spray large nonstick skillet with cooking spray; heat over medium-high heat. Add mushrooms; cook 4 minutes or until mushrooms are soft, stirring frequently. Transfer to pie plate. Add broccoli to skillet; cook and stir 2 minutes. Transfer to pie plate with mushrooms.

3. Whisk egg substitute, milk, salt, thyme and red pepper in medium bowl. Stir until well blended. Stir in green onions and ¾ cup cheese. Pour evenly over vegetable mixture. Bake 25 to 30 minutes or until knife inserted in center comes out clean.

4. Remove from oven. Sprinkle evenly with remaining ¼ cup cheese. Let stand 10 minutes before cutting into quarters.

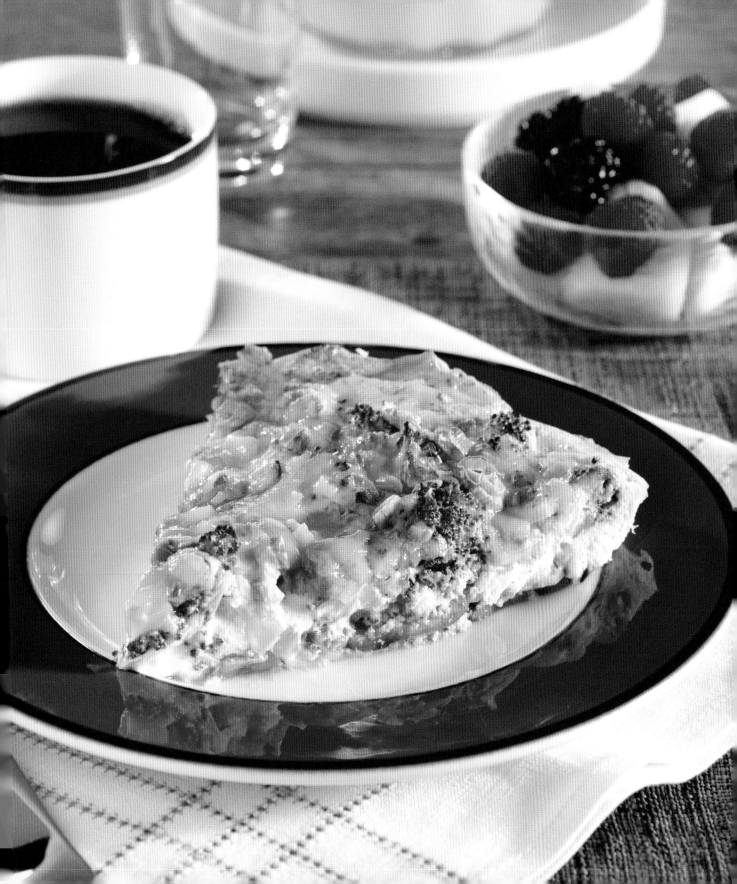

Smoked Salmon
and Spinach Frittata

makes 6 servings

PER SERVING

330 **calories**
23g **total fat**
3g **carbs**
2g **net carbs**
1g **dietary fiber**
23g **protein**

2 tablespoons olive oil, divided

1 medium red onion, diced

1 clove garlic, minced

6 ounces baby spinach

10 eggs

1 teaspoon dried dill weed

¼ teaspoon salt

¼ teaspoon black pepper

4 ounces smoked salmon, chopped

4 ounces aged Cheddar cheese, cut into ¼-inch cubes

1. Position oven rack in upper-middle position. Preheat broiler.

2. Heat 1 tablespoon oil in large ovenproof nonstick skillet. Add onion; cook 7 to 8 minutes or until softened, stirring occasionally. Add garlic; cook and stir 1 minute. Add spinach; cook and stir 3 minutes or just until wilted. Transfer mixture to small bowl.

3. Whisk eggs, dill, salt and pepper in large bowl until blended. Stir in salmon, cheese and spinach mixture.

4. Heat remaining 1 tablespoon oil in same skillet over medium heat. Add egg mixture; cook about 3 minutes, stirring gently to form large curds. Cook without stirring 5 minutes or until eggs are just beginning to set.

5. Transfer skillet to oven. Broil 2 to 3 minutes or until frittata is puffed, set and lightly browned. Let stand 5 minutes; carefully slide frittata onto large plate or cutting board. Cut into wedges.

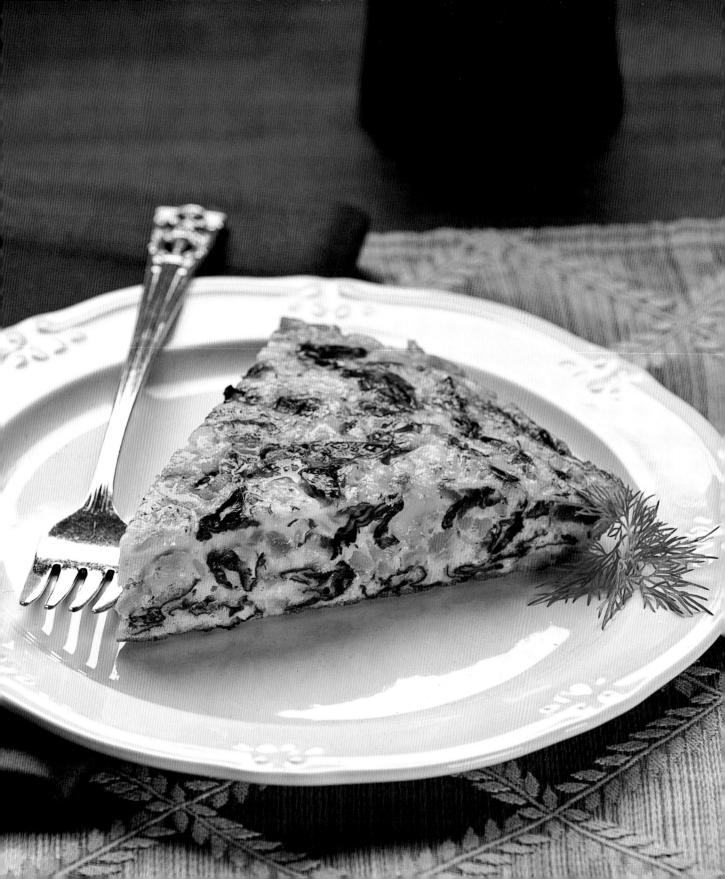

Everything Bagels

makes 12 bagels

PER SERVING

210 **calories**
19 **total fat**
5 **carbs**
3 **net carbs**
2 **dietary fiber**
8 **protein**

6 eggs, at room temperature, separated

¼ teaspoon cream of tartar

2 cups almond flour

3½ teaspoons baking powder

½ teaspoon salt

¼ teaspoon garlic powder

6 tablespoons butter, melted and cooled slightly

½ cup finely shredded Asiago cheese

2 tablespoons everything bagel seasoning

1. Preheat oven to 350°F. Spray 12 cavities of doughnut pans with nonstick cooking spray.

2. Place egg whites and cream of tartar in large bowl; attach whisk attachment to stand mixer. Whip egg whites on high speed 2 minutes or until stiff peaks form. Transfer egg whites to medium bowl.

3. Combine almond flour, baking powder, salt and garlic powder in mixer bowl. Add melted butter and egg yolks; mix on medium speed until well blended. Add cheese; mix well.

4. Stir one third of egg whites into almond flour mixture with spatula until well blended. Gently fold in remaining egg whites until thoroughly blended. Scoop mixture into large resealable food storage bag; cut off one corner. Pipe about ¼ cup batter into each doughnut cavity. Sprinkle each with ½ teaspoon everything bagel seasoning.

5. Bake about 10 minutes or until bagels are golden brown and set. Cool in pans 2 minutes. Remove to wire rack; serve warm or cool completely.

Everything Bagel Muffins: If you don't have doughnut pans or would prefer to make muffins instead, scoop batter into 12 greased standard muffin pan cups. Sprinkle with bagel seasoning. Bake 15 minutes or until tops are golden brown and toothpick inserted into centers comes out clean.

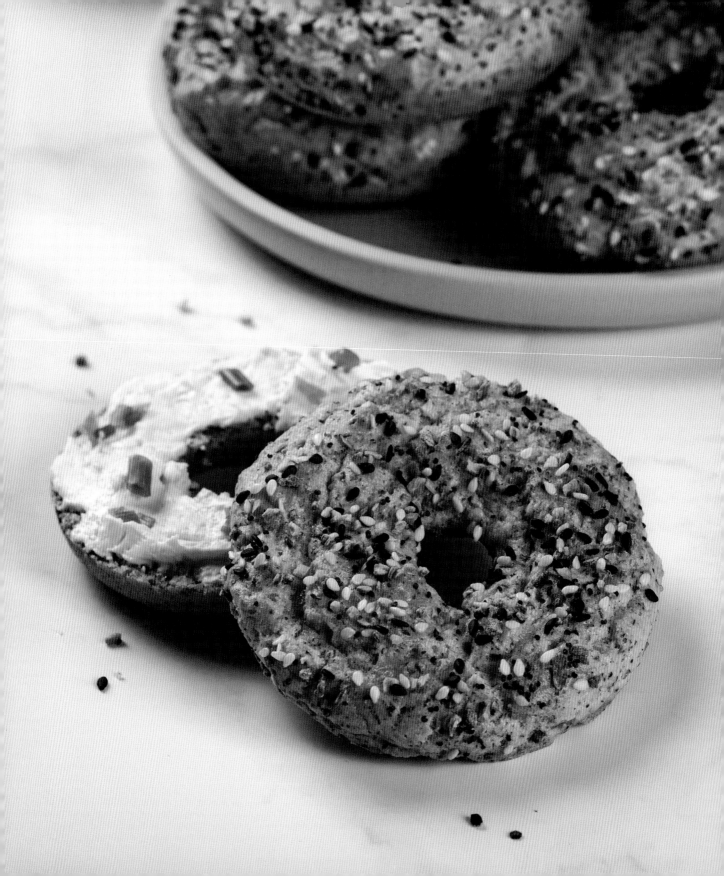

Mediterranean Frittata

makes 6 servings

¼ cup extra virgin olive oil

5 small onions, thinly sliced

1 can (about 14 ounces) whole tomatoes, drained and chopped

4 ounces prosciutto or cooked ham, chopped

¼ cup grated Parmesan cheese

2 tablespoons chopped fresh parsley

½ teaspoon dried marjoram

¼ teaspoon salt

¼ teaspoon dried basil

⅛ teaspoon black pepper

6 eggs

2 tablespoons butter

1. Heat oil in large skillet over medium-high heat. Add onions; cook and stir 8 to 10 minutes until soft and golden. Reduce heat to medium. Add tomatoes; cook 5 minutes. Remove vegetables to large bowl with slotted spoon; discard drippings. Cool to room temperature.

2. Stir prosciutto, Parmesan, parsley, marjoram, salt, basil and pepper into tomato mixture. Whisk eggs in medium bowl; stir into prosciutto mixture.

3. Preheat broiler. Heat butter in medium ovenproof skillet over medium heat until melted and bubbly. Reduce heat to low; add egg mixture to skillet, spreading evenly. Cook 8 to 10 minutes until all but top ¼ inch of frittata is set. (Shake pan gently to test.) *Do not stir.*

4. Broil frittata about 4 inches from heat 1 to 2 minutes or until top is set. (Do not brown or frittata will be dry.) Serve warm or at room temperature. Cut into wedges.

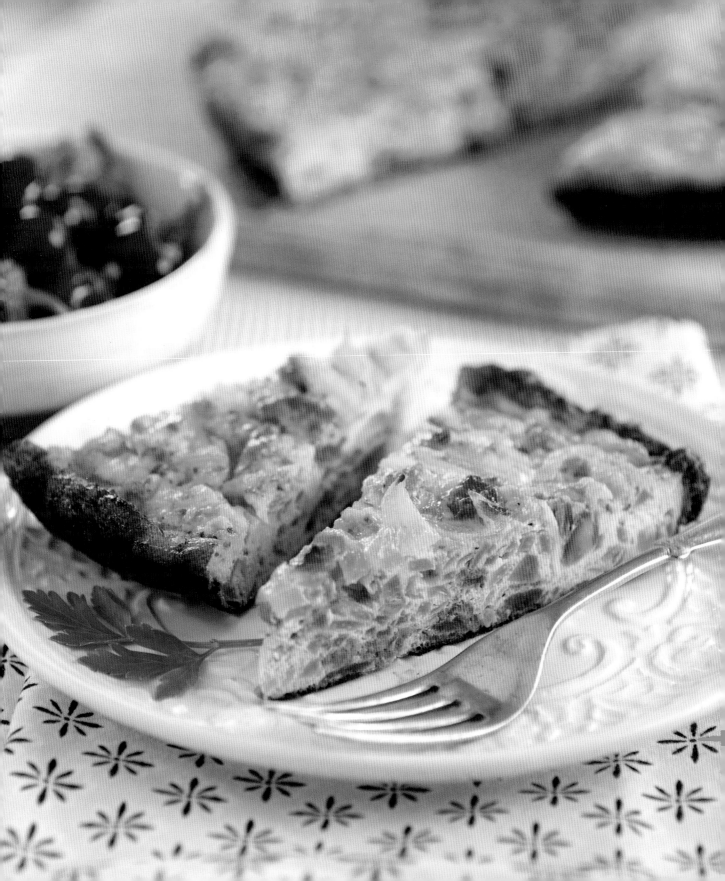

metric conversion chart

VOLUME MEASUREMENTS (dry)

$1/8$ teaspoon = 0.5 mL
$1/4$ teaspoon = 1 mL
$1/2$ teaspoon = 2 mL
$3/4$ teaspoon = 4 mL
1 teaspoon = 5 mL
1 tablespoon = 15 mL
2 tablespoons = 30 mL
$1/4$ cup = 60 mL
$1/3$ cup = 75 mL
$1/2$ cup = 125 mL
$2/3$ cup = 150 mL
$3/4$ cup = 175 mL
1 cup = 250 mL
2 cups = 1 pint = 500 mL
3 cups = 750 mL
4 cups = 1 quart = 1 L

VOLUME MEASUREMENTS (fluid)

1 fluid ounce (2 tablespoons) = 30 mL
4 fluid ounces ($1/2$ cup) = 125 mL
8 fluid ounces (1 cup) = 250 mL
12 fluid ounces ($1 1/2$ cups) = 375 mL
16 fluid ounces (2 cups) = 500 mL

WEIGHTS (mass)

$1/2$ ounce = 15 g
1 ounce = 30 g
3 ounces = 90 g
4 ounces = 120 g
8 ounces = 225 g
10 ounces = 285 g
12 ounces = 360 g
16 ounces = 1 pound = 450 g

DIMENSIONS

$1/16$ inch = 2 mm
$1/8$ inch = 3 mm
$1/4$ inch = 6 mm
$1/2$ inch = 1.5 cm
$3/4$ inch = 2 cm
1 inch = 2.5 cm

OVEN TEMPERATURES

250°F = 120°C
275°F = 140°C
300°F = 150°C
325°F = 160°C
350°F = 180°C
375°F = 190°C
400°F = 200°C
425°F = 220°C
450°F = 230°C

BAKING PAN SIZES

Utensil	Size in Inches/Quarts	Metric Volume	Size in Centimeters
Baking or Cake Pan (square or rectangular)	$8\times8\times2$	2 L	$20\times20\times5$
	$9\times9\times2$	2.5 L	$23\times23\times5$
	$12\times8\times2$	3 L	$30\times20\times5$
	$13\times9\times2$	3.5 L	$33\times23\times5$
Loaf Pan	$8\times4\times3$	1.5 L	$20\times10\times7$
	$9\times5\times3$	2 L	$23\times13\times7$
Round Layer Cake Pan	$8\times1 1/2$	1.2 L	20×4
	$9\times1 1/2$	1.5 L	23×4
Pie Plate	$8\times1 1/4$	750 mL	20×3
	$9\times1 1/4$	1 L	23×3
Baking Dish or Casserole	1 quart	1 L	—
	$1 1/2$ quart	1.5 L	—
	2 quart	2 L	—